MW01137702

Unplug

HOW TO BREAK UP
WITH YOUR PHONE AND
RECLAIM YOUR LIFE

RICHARD SIMON

WORKMAN PUBLISHING | NEW YORK

Workman
Workman Publishing
Hachette Book Group, Inc.
1290 Avenue of the Americas
New York, NY 10104
workman.com

Workman is an imprint of Workman Publishing, a division of Hachette Book Group, Inc. The Workman name and logo are registered trademarks of Hachette Book Group, Inc.

Design by Jack Dunnington and Galen Smith
Author photo by Brent Futrell

Workman books may be purchased in bulk for business, educational, or promotional use. For information, please contact your local bookseller or the Hachette Book Group Special Markets Department at special.markets@hbgusa.com.

Library of Congress Cataloging-in-Publication Data is available.

ISBN: 978-1-5235-2756-4

First Edition June 2025

Printed in China on responsibly sourced paper.

10 9 8 7 6 5 4 3 2 1

To Lauren

Contents

Introduction

In February 2021, Nick Castellanos drove across the country from his home in South Florida to his team's spring training complex outside of Phoenix, Arizona.

A right fielder for the Cincinnati Reds, Castellanos was entering his ninth year in the majors. One of the top prospects coming out of the 2010 draft, he spent most of his career in the Detroit Tigers organization before being traded to the Chicago Cubs, then landing a four-year deal with the Reds.

Like many players whose routines were upended by the coronavirus pandemic, Castellanos had a down year in the shortened 2020 season, setting a career low in batting average. During the offseason, the twenty-eight-year-old took time to reflect, thinking about his life, his profession, and his relationships with his soon-to-be wife, son, parents, and teammates. One of the sticking points that ran through all his reflections was his smartphone.

"I knew what I wanted, but I had no idea what to do about it," he told me.

He found himself lost in the addictive nature of the device—the group chats, videos of baseball swings, funny memes, fantasy football, and viral videos.

During a season, he would frequently read baseball news, both good and bad, including critiques of how he was playing. He would read the analysis of who swung this way and that, who was hot and who was not.

He tried deleting social media apps to improve his relationship with his iPhone, but it wasn't enough. It led to a realization.

"If I really wanted to be the best baseball player I can be, have the marriage I want to have, the father I want to be, son, brother and friend . . . I needed to get rid of it."

After completing his physical upon arrival at the Reds' spring training facility, he sat down that evening by a fire and wrote down on a piece of paper:

Either I will continue to try and understand the universe or the universe will try to understand me.

It was at that point that Castellanos turned off his smartphone, opting for a flip phone instead. Rather than keep his old phone number, Castellanos decided to "start from scratch."

The original idea was to turn it off for the entire baseball season, eight months if you count spring training.

"Let's bubble up and focus on this baseball season," he told himself. "Let's get my shit in order and let's lock it in."

Castellanos would quickly learn that flipping the switch wasn't so easy. The first week was rocky. He felt anxious without the device by his side and missed the alluring ease of anything being a swipe away. Nevertheless, he adjusted.

During spring training, he developed a focus on the field that he hadn't experienced before in his career, from his training with box jumps to his ability to get in the zone at the plate. He felt more disciplined and committed with each at bat; he was no longer letting himself deviate or allowing someone else's negative energy interfere with what he wanted to do.

"The game improved because I had a much clearer mind, focus, and awareness. I was a more engaged baseball player," he said.

. . . . .

On Opening Day of the 2021 season, Castellanos went three for five with a home run against the St. Louis Cardinals. In his second game, he was hit by a pitch in the fourth inning by Cardinals pitcher Jake Woodford and later scored on a wild pitch, sliding into home plate headfirst as Woodward fell on top of him trying to tag him out. Afterward, he popped up, yelled, and flexed his muscles over Woodford as the pitcher lay on the ground, leading to both benches clearing.

Castellanos was suspended for two games for instigating, but the image of him pumping his muscles would become what *Cincinnati Enquirer* baseball writer Bobby Nightengale called "a rallying cry throughout the city." A billboard was even erected outside of the Reds' stadium to capture the moment.

Castellanos's stellar play continued. During the first half of the season, he mashed for a major-league best .346 batting average and led the league in hits and doubles. He was voted to his first All-Star Game and selected as the starting right fielder for the National League.

"He played as well as the Reds could have dreamed of. He became a team leader, and everything came together," Nightengale said.

Castellanos hit .309 for the season and tallied thirty-four home runs, both career highs. He won his first Silver Slugger Award, an honor bestowed by Major League Baseball's managers and coaches to the best offensive player at each position.

Castellanos is convinced that turning off his smartphone was one of the biggest factors in his success on the field. As we spoke more, he explained how other areas of his life had improved off the field as well.

He began a nighttime ritual at his home in Cincinnati that included putting on relaxing music and sitting by an outdoor fire. Without the distraction of technology, including the barrage of messages he'd usually receive after games, Castellanos said the sounds of the piano and the crackling fire would allow him to reflect after a busy day on the field.

"I was just being," he explained.

By focusing on his own personal well-being, he had more energy for other areas of his life, including spending time with his wife, son, and friends.

Before the 2021 season, Castellanos would often text with his teammates in group chats. When I asked him what his teammates thought of his decision to get rid of his smartphone, he told me, "Everybody on the team 100 percent thinks I'm crazy. But I don't mind it . . . because now the conversations that I have with my teammates . . . are meaningful ones, talking about the game, talking about our team, talking about how we're doing."

With a flip phone, Castellanos explained, "texting is a nightmare." He has to punch numbers multiple times to find the right letter, causing enough frustration to eliminate what he identified as "meaningless conversation."

"I enjoy talking to people now," he said.

I asked Castellanos if he ever got burned by not having a smartphone. He paused for a moment. "I have one [story]," he offered.

After a road game, he went back to the team's hotel and was starving. It was after midnight and room service was no longer available. "I couldn't Uber Eats anything . . . and I was really frustrated for about ten minutes, and then I was like, 'what a beautiful opportunity to practice being hungry.'"

I was amazed. An entire season without a smartphone and the only low point he could think of was not being able to pull off online food delivery.

When I spoke to Castellanos for the first time, it was three weeks after his remarkable 2021 season had ended—and he still hadn't turned back on his smartphone.

It Doesn't Have to Be This Way

Over a two-year period, I had dozens of conversations with Castellanos and others who recognized the challenges that can come with owning a smartphone and decided to do something about it.

If you picked up a copy of this book, you're probably in the early stages of wanting to develop a healthier relationship with your smartphone. And though just about everyone has good intentions when they purchase a phone, more and more of us are realizing that we're spending far too much time on them.

"If we feel 'addicted to our phones,' it is not a personal weakness. We are exhibiting a predictable response to a perfectly executed design," writes MIT professor Sherry Turkle in her book *Reclaiming Conversation*.

You likely wanted all that modern smartphones can deliver: You looked forward to easily accessing the internet, making calls and sending text messages on the go, sending out work emails from home or on your commute, streaming Netflix, capturing and storing photos, reading the news, using social media, listening to your favorite podcast, keeping track of your fitness, playing video games during down time, monitoring stocks, getting directions—the list gets bigger with each new phone iteration.

But with this easy access comes a dark side for many of us: a constant state of distraction.

New York University professor of marketing Adam Alter writes in his book *Irresistible*, "We shouldn't use a watered-down term to describe them [smartphones]. We should acknowledge how serious they are, how much harm they're doing to our collective well-being, and how much attention they deserve. The evidence so far is concerning, and trends suggest we're wading deeper into dangerous waters."

Dr. Anna Lembke, a Stanford University professor of psychiatry, calls the smartphone "the modern-day hypodermic needle, delivering digital dopamine for a wired generation."

If you're using it unchecked, your smartphone might be stealing your attention away from being with family or reducing your ability to concentrate on work and tasks. You might feel relationships are suffering or you just can't slow life down. You might have forgotten what it means to experience solitude, to be alone with your thoughts.

If any of these concerns ring a bell, I was in the same position as you.

As a thirty-three-year-old father of two in 2019, spending hours each day on my smartphone, I felt helpless. I tried so many different hacks recommended in self-help articles to form a more effective relationship with my phone, but none of them got me to my end goal of being in control of it rather than it being in control of me.

I came to realize that my smartphone had existential implications. There are so many facets of life we don't understand, yet one undeniable truth persists: Time is a finite resource. Meaning, one day each one of us will die.

I realized that I was spending hours each day on my smartphone—time that I couldn't get back.

The average American spends more than five hours a day on their smartphone—that means more than a quarter of our waking hours are spent on the devices. Most teenagers spend half their waking hours on them.

This is the moment to take a stand. You *can* reset the relationship you have with your phone. It is time to stop wasting time—and reclaim it.

Consider this book a manifesto. In the pages that follow, I propose a new vision for how to use your phone.

You will learn how important it is to do a proper smartphone detox. That means turning it off to recalibrate the reward pathways in your brain. I will offer a slew of real-life examples of people who underwent detoxes, illustrating the different approaches they took.

With hours of newfound time, I'll point out areas of your life you can improve. We'll consider what the reintegration phase looks like if you decide to turn your smartphone back on, as well as the importance of speaking to others about your journey.

All of the strategies I offer are supported by real-life examples and established science, as well as the opinions of leading addiction specialists and subject matter experts.

Among others, you'll be introduced to an anesthesiologist in Baltimore, a software engineer in Seattle, a social media marketer in Northern Ireland, a school principal in Chicago, and a law partner in Connecticut. There's also a writer in Vermont, a product specialist in Kenya, a college senior at the University of Notre Dame, a chess grand master in Minnesota, and a financial analyst in Italy—all of whom fundamentally changed their relationships with their phones and enhanced their lives in remarkable ways.

You will find that living a better life with your phone isn't exclusive to any one person or lifestyle—it is something that can work for everyone.

I approach this topic with a great sense of humility. Like most people, I'm trying to figure out the world and advance my life in positive ways. So, you might be wondering, why me? Why is Richard Simon, a relative unknown, writing this book?

Because I'm all of you. I was sick and tired of my smartphone taking away from the quality of my life and I did something about it. I wanted to further my goals, my hopes and dreams for myself and my family—and I firmly believe you can too.

If there's one thing that I can say after my journey of quitting my smartphone and talking to dozens and dozens of people who did the same, it is this: You have control over your life. You can decide how you spend your time. Just because everyone is looking down at their phones on the train or tapping away across from you at dinner, it doesn't mean you have to do the same. The power is in your hands.

When you follow the advice in this book, you aren't just going to break up with your phone, you will also become a better version of yourself.

Let's begin the journey.

CHAPTER 1

A Year Without a Smartphone

In the summer of 2017, Robert Hassan had an awakening. A professor at the University of Melbourne in Australia, Hassan taught media and communications, focusing much of his scholarship on the study of time.

Yet for many years, he didn't reflect on his own relationship with digital technology, and how he was losing control of time. Until one day, at the age of fifty-eight, he did.

He began to account for all of the time he spent on his smartphone, distractedly surfing websites, like so many of us do.

"I thought I was immune to that kind of thing," Hassan told me. "But in fact, I wasn't. The time you take looking at the screen is time you don't get back. The way the internet is set up is to attract you, distract you, and to keep you clicking through website after website."

Hassan's daily bike ride to the university would take him past Swanson dock, a container-shipping terminal. As he was wrestling internally with his digital habits, he started to fantasize what it might be like to go on a container ship, to be isolated, to unplug.

One evening at home, he discovered that container ships allow a small number of passengers on board. Even better, there was a ship leaving in several days from Swanson dock on a five-week journey from Melbourne to Singapore.

On a whim, and without a research grant or university funding, Hassan signed the mandatory waivers and paperwork and purchased a passenger ticket for the CMA CGM *Rossini*.

To make it a true digital detox, Hassan went minimal with what he brought on board. Notable items he packed included six notebooks, a box of pencils, a pencil sharpener, five books, and a Swiss Army knife.

With only a few crew members aboard who spoke English, Hassan spent most of his time in his cabin, which had a window view, or he walked around the ship, embracing the sounds of the ocean and its vast expanse.

"I had the chance to go deeper than I ever had gone before," he told me. "Being isolated the way I was, I found that I started to look more inward, and at my own memories. Something which we can all do when we have the time, but we mostly don't."

With little to do around the ship, he put his Swiss Army knife to use by disassembling a chair in his room and putting it back together. He also thought more intensely about the meaning of time, keeping a daily journal of his experiences. Without an alarm clock, he experienced triphasic sleep, waking up in the middle of the night, being active for a couple of hours before going back to sleep again with a nap midday. Sleep, as he found it, in its most natural form.

Hassan would later document the digital detox in his book *Uncontained*.

. . . . .

When I spoke to him in the fall of 2021, four years after his voyage, I wanted to know whether he had changed because of the experience.

"I've become a different person," he told me. "I've become a person who is more self-aware and self-knowing. I learned things about myself through the deep dive of memory that I didn't know. I feel I gave myself depth in terms of my consciousness, my being. I felt grateful for that."

Hassan explained that his craftsmanship on the vessel inspired him to do more work with his hands. During the coronavirus pandemic, he learned how to repair watches as a hobby. He also continued his triphasic sleep pattern, as well as journaling, which allows him to process his thoughts.

Hassan's digital detox inspired me. When I first read his story on bestselling author Cal Newport's blog in 2019, it got me thinking about what I could do to reclaim my own life.

The idea of turning off your devices to connect on a deeper level with the world made me envious. Like so many of us, I had an unhealthy relationship with my smartphone. My phone habits had been bothering me for years. I can't pinpoint when it became a problem, but over time I came to realize I was living a less meaningful life because of my phone.

My Story of Digital Distraction

I used a basic phone for the first few years after the original iPhone was released in 2007. This was partly for financial reasons—as a college senior I couldn't justify the added expense, and after graduation, my job as a reporter at a daily newspaper in Baltimore didn't require it.

But when I started working for Georgetown Law in Washington, DC, managing their website in 2010, I quickly realized that most of my colleagues had smartphones and were using them throughout the day. They checked them during meetings, refreshing their inboxes with a quick swipe of the thumb. They would bring them to lunch, setting them on the table next to their food. Outside of work, my friends were doing what felt new at the time: capturing and sharing photos and communicating using apps.

Smartphones were becoming ubiquitous, and I was feeling more and more like an outsider without one, like I didn't belong. The social pressure to get one was mounting. Eventually, I gave in and made the leap, purchasing an iPhone 3GS in January 2011. The day after I bought it, I remember going on a date. We were at a pizza shop, sitting across from each other in a booth, as I excitedly showed her all the phone's cool features.

I didn't understand it at the time, but just about all aspects of my life would soon be affected by this tiny device.

"Basic" Phone vs. Smartphone

* A basic phone is a cell phone used primarily to call and text. It may also be referred to as a flip phone, brick phone, or dumbphone.

* A smartphone is closer to a minicomputer with additional functionality that includes internet access, email, apps (including social media), and advanced camera specifications, among other features.

FROM CELL PHONE TO SMARTPHONE: A STUDY IN UBIQUITY

Motorola chief executive Martin Cooper made history in 1973 when he used a DynaTAC 8000X to make the world's first public call with a portable, handheld cell phone that measured ten inches long and nearly two and a half pounds. And the world, as they say, would never be the same.

Even before the iPhone's inception in 2007, the cell phone was a transformative device. According to a 2005 Pew report, the majority of Americans under the age of sixty-five owned a cell phone. A 2006 Pew study found that 52 percent of cell phone users never turned off their phones, with 41 percent of people saying they made phone calls to fill time while waiting for something or while traveling.

At the turn of the twenty-first century, smartphones like the Blackberry and Palm Treo became popular, especially as part of work, with immediate access to internet and email.

Gerard Goggin is an internationally renowned scholar on mobile technology who has been tracking the history of the cell phone and its use for decades. In his 2006 book *Cell Phone Culture*, released one year before the creation of the iPhone, he catalogs many of the anxieties that people had regarding overuse of the device, with teens in particular spending excessive amounts of time texting.

He also noted that the cell phone aided mass movements at the beginning of the twenty-first century, including the Arab Spring and the overthrow of various governments. In 2001, for example, text messages spurred over a million protesters to gather in Manila to oust Filipino president Joseph Estrada.

And then came the watershed moment in 2007.

When Steve Jobs introduced the iPhone to a captivated audience at the Moscone Center in San Francisco, he introduced the ability to not only call and text, but also to seamlessly surf the internet, read email, take pictures, stream video, check stocks, listen to music or podcasts, add items to your calendar, write notes, and more. The smartphone was unlike any other technology that preceded it in its portability and amalgamation, and that was even before social media apps were introduced.

The multitouch user interface that allowed for swiping and pinching was created by some of the top designers in the world who set out to make even the most mundane interactions feel compelling.

Inspired by video games, the designers of the iPhone created an experience that makes you want to keep using it.

Incredible care and attention was given to each individual icon and swipe.

When one of the lead iPhone designers tested the slide-to-unlock function on his baby daughter and was successful, the team knew it worked.

Shockingly, for one of the most transformative devices in modern life, there were only twenty to twenty-five people who worked on the iPhone in its development.

Apple's iPhone team worked in an abandoned user-testing facility, a space where no usability testing was actually done on the iPhone.

"Steve Jobs really didn't believe in user testing," said Brian Merchant, who wrote *The One Device: The Secret History of the iPhone*. "He thought it was worthless, his whole maxim was, we're going to tell the user what they want and then they're gonna like it."

Steve Krug, a user-testing expert, told me that he was once hired by Apple to teach a usability testing workshop about five years after the release of the iPhone.

"One of the most interesting things to me working with this group of developers and designers was they immediately said, 'Our problem is we can't show it [our work] to anybody.'"

The development of the iPhone was so secretive that even the cleaning crews weren't allowed in the workspace.

After the release of the iPhone, using a smartphone became more and more commonplace. In 2011, one-third of Americans said they used a smartphone. By 2024, nine in ten Americans had one. For ages 18–49, ownership was 97 percent.

Looking past its ubiquity, and additional features that have been added to the iPhone over the years including the App Store and an improved camera, the core iPhone we hold today still looks very much the same as it did in 2007. The icons for Safari, Email, and Messages still greet us the same way they did close to two decades ago.

And the core problem that its release created in 2007 remains the same today: It has redefined our daily lives in how much time we spend on them.

When Merchant interviewed the key players involved in the design and development of the iPhone a decade ago, he was surprised to find a near-universal ambivalence. Most were awed by the reach of the device, but also by the downsides of its constant distraction.

"They talked about going to restaurants and seeing everybody buried in their phones and the dampening effect that put on the ability for people to have sort of normal social experiences and communication. . . . I think they were grappling then with the most immediate effects," recalled Merchant.

Pre-smartphone, when I traveled on the MARC commuter train from my home in Baltimore to work in Washington, DC, I read books. On the hour-long train ride, I focused intensely, becoming a prolific reader. But with my shiny new iPhone, with internet surfing and music streaming a tap away, I didn't feel as much of a need to bring books on the train. If I had a moment of silence, I would quickly reach for my phone to fill the void.

Instead of calling friends, we texted. My dating relationships would start off on text, and in most cases continue over text between dates. I would check my phone incessantly throughout the day to see if a new text had come through.

I had difficulty focusing on tasks at the office, with a notification or ding constantly shifting my attention, the distraction inevitably impacting the quality of my work.

I woke up in the morning with my phone by my side and went to bed checking it with the lights off. I brought it with me into the bathroom. At synagogue during daily prayer services, I had my prayer book in one hand, and would often reach for my cell phone to hold in the other. On the golf course, I placed it in my golf bag and would check it between shots.

At first, I thought this addictive behavior was rare. That I was an outlier. But soon after I married my wife, Lauren, and we were preparing for our first child in 2016, I started to look around more. I gazed up and down the train station waiting area in the morning and realized that most people were looking down at their phones. On the train itself, even if a person was asleep there were usually headphones involved. At concerts, people looked at their phones while recording the musicians on stage instead of actually watching them with their own eyes.

I soon realized that I wasn't alone, that something else was going on. At baseball games, I couldn't find anyone near me who wasn't context switching between their phone and the game. On walks around the neighborhood, when most people should be getting away from technology, most people I saw were either looking down at their phones or streaming music. At dinner with friends, it became difficult to have conversations with people, with a ding or vibration at the table abruptly ending whatever was being discussed.

.....

Once kids came into the picture—Akiva in 2016 and Hillel in 2019—I knew something had to change. I started to try different methods to become less dependent on my phone.

Digital sabbaths had become a popular method to disconnect one day a week. As a Sabbath-observant Orthodox Jew, I was very familiar with this method and found the twenty-four hours from sundown Friday to sundown Saturday to be a sacred and restorative time.

I would feel such relief when I turned off my phone Friday evenings, a weight lifted off my shoulders. No work emails to check, no text messages coming through, just time to reconnect with family and friends.

But once late afternoon arrived on Saturday, several hours before the completion of the Sabbath, I would start to feel the dopamine rush, the anticipation of turning on my phone to check for messages and see what news I'd missed over the last twenty-four hours. After we'd extinguish the flame of the Havdalah candle, I'd rush from the kitchen to our bedroom to turn on my phone, eager to see what I had missed.

Turning my phone off for the Sabbath was a Band-Aid, I realized, like telling someone who is addicted to cigarettes not to smoke for one day a week. I knew it wouldn't solve my problem.

I experimented with leaving my phone in the mudroom when I got back from work and keeping it there for the remainder of the evening. If I had to check something I'd walk over, tap my phone, complete my task, and then leave. The inconvenience of not having it by my side made me feel less dependent on it at home, but also showed me how dangerous a tool it was.

I would often wonder what my oldest son was thinking every half hour when I would leave the game or puzzle we were working on to check my phone by the carport door, hearing the latest ding, or giving in to the urge to refresh my email inbox. I felt like I had an addiction to a drug, picking up our youngest son with one arm after changing a diaper and walking to the other side of our house to check my phone with the other hand. It felt wrong.

I tried turning on airplane mode and deleting applications. But on stroller walks around the neighborhood, I'd still tap my phone to see the time, look at my calendar, and open my email and messages even if I knew new messages weren't going to come in. The mere motion of tapping my phone and the shining light coming on was so ingrained in my routine.

As I know now, what I was trying were just "hacks" (see page 49). Noble as they might have been, these efforts didn't get me close enough to what I was looking for.

I knew the relationship with my wife, Lauren, was suffering from how much time I was spending on my smartphone. I spent hours on it each day, especially in the evening—time that could have been spent with her. I felt that I wasn't able to focus on Akiva and Hillel as much as I wanted to. Trips to the zoo and aquarium felt distracted. The kids' morning and afternoon naps, when I could have been productive, were instead spent on the sofa looking at my phone.

Digital Hacks vs. Digital Detox

- Digital Hack: A technique for reducing the problematic effects of a specific behavior, but not entirely.
- Digital Detox: The process of disconnecting completely from a substance that is unhealthy, in this case, a smartphone.

I had been working at Georgetown Law for nine years, and I felt that I wasn't gaining as much in career capital as I'd like, largely because I couldn't focus deeply. I also wasn't finding the time to invest in meaningful activities, such as reading, writing, and golf.

And then there was me. I didn't have time for self-reflection. I couldn't embrace solitude. During any quiet moment, I would seek out my phone. While waiting in line at the grocery store, I took it out. At a baseball game, I would check it frequently to see if a message had come in. It was a pacifier, a way to escape the realities of life. I lost who I was, who I wanted to be.

It's why Robert Hassan's story of riding on a container ship was so powerful to me. After I read it, I knew I needed to do something drastic, though maybe not something quite so radical.

I had another idea. It was November, two months shy of 2020. In January, I wanted to turn off my smartphone—for an entire year.

WHY SMARTPHONES ARE SO ADDICTIVE

Why is it that the average American unlocks their phone 150 times a day? How is it possible that at any given time, more than 800,000 drivers are using a handheld cell phone during daylight hours? What makes our phones so addictive, so pervasively difficult to resist?

The leading culprit is one of the most powerful molecules in the brain: dopamine.

Each time you reach for your phone and tap the screen, your brain releases dopamine. The release of dopamine is pleasurable, and your brain will crave more. This reinforces the behavior of checking your phone throughout the day.

There is an excitement and unpredictability of not knowing what you are going to see when you open up your phone. Will there be new text messages? Did a work colleague respond to your most recent email? What will the latest news alert be?

"That is the dopamine process at work," said Dr. Mike Brooks, a psychologist based out of Austin, Texas, who specializes in screens and technology. "Dopamine isn't just like a one-trick pony. Once you get into a habit of checking your phone, the dopamine incentivizes you to check the phone. It creates an itch that needs to get scratched."

Because of how little friction there is to getting each dopamine hit—from unlocking your phone to tapping on an icon—each interaction is rewarded.

"Crack cocaine was much more addictive than regular cocaine because of a very short difference in time it took people to get high," said Dr. Clifford Sussman, a screen addiction specialist with a private practice in Washington, DC. "In the case of a smartphone . . . it's basically a shortcut machine and nothing is more powerful for the reward system of your brain than a shortcut machine."

NYU marketing professor Adam Alter explains that behavioral addictions embody at least one of the following six ingredients:

- Compelling goals that are just beyond reach
- Irresistible and unpredictable positive feedback
- A sense of incremental progress and improvement
- Tasks that become slowly more difficult over time
- Unresolved tensions that demand resolution
- Strong social connections

"Addictions bring the promise of immediate reward, or positive reinforcement," he explains.

There is also a feeling of power when it comes to using our phones.

Rachel Plotnick, a professor at Indiana University Bloomington who studies human-machine relationships, including our interaction with interfaces, found that control and agency are fundamental to why phones make us feel powerful, and why they're pleasurable and desirable.

"People feel like they're in control when they're pushing buttons, and not only is that a dopamine effect, but it's also a powerful feeling," she said. "That's why when you put people in an elevator with no buttons, they will freak out and have panic attacks because they don't like the idea of being in a steel box where they don't get to control the machine."

The Conversation

I first pitched the idea to Lauren. To say she was less than thrilled would be an understatement. Lauren is a pediatrician, and a darn good one. Like any doctor would do, she ran through the potential scenarios where my idea wouldn't work.

- What if I'm out with our three-year-old son, Akiva, and he has another anaphylactic reaction to tree nuts and has to be taken to the hospital?

- What if something happened to our six-month-old son, Hillel, and I'm at work and she can't get in touch with me?

- What if there is an emergency at school?

- What if there is a terrorist attack on the train? (This was a real scenario we played out.)

- How will I know you got safely to work?

Eventually, I made an emotional plea: "I want to reconnect with you."

It was true. When I first met Lauren she was in her second year of medical school and I was commuting from Baltimore to Washington every day during the week. Finding time to spend together was hard.

After we got married, the two of us would plop down on the sofa in the living room after a long day of work. We would sit there for an hour, sometimes two, often with our smartphones in hand. As I know now, we weren't really together. Together is when we look into each other's eyes, not at a screen.

So much of the communication in our relationship was centered on texting. To the point that when we both got back from work, there wasn't anything to catch up on. We had already told each other everything over text during the day.

Yet what I really wanted to say at that moment was selfish. I didn't say it, though I probably should have: I also wanted to reconnect with me.

At thirty-three, I felt like I was losing out on life. So many wasted days and nights mindlessly spent on a device that gave me more anxiety than happiness. I wasn't growing as a father or a person in the ways I hoped.

I knew that in life, as I mentioned earlier, time is a finite resource. And I was never going to get back the hours I spent each day on my phone. I wanted to move forward in life, but I was remaining stagnant.

A day after I proposed the one-year detox, out of the goodness of her heart, Lauren gave me her blessing, and said I could do it. I hugged her, trying to hold in my excitement.

"You won't regret this."

As I let go of the embrace, I saw the skeptical look on her face. I understood that turning off my smartphone would impact her as well.

Days later, after thinking through the project more, hoping to give Lauren some peace of mind, I decided that I would follow two simple ground rules:

1. I wasn't going to throw my smartphone away. In fact, in some cases, I would bring my smartphone with me when I left the house. If there was ever an emergency, I would use it. That meant that I would take it with me to work, or on activities with the boys, but I would always leave it off.

2. Just because my phone was turned off didn't mean that I could use hers, or someone else's. No cheating.

I was excited to turn off my phone, but also nervous. How would I tell my boss at work that I wouldn't be using my phone for a year? As a technology professional directing the website strategy for one of the top law schools in the country, it was paramount that I be available, especially during the two days a week I worked from home when I felt like I needed to be more connected.

On the train, I would often respond to emails that came in at the end of the day. Even on weekends or days off, I would try to stay on top of messages coming in with my phone. I prided myself on my level of responsiveness.

Then there were friends. How would my relationships with them be impacted? I communicated over text a lot. What would happen to people who texted me and I never got their messages? Would they find another way to get in touch, or would the relationships suffer?

What I decided was risky. I made the decision to not tell anyone what I was doing (as you'll read in the next chapter, don't follow this logic!). Not my colleagues, not my closest friends. Lauren knew, of course, and I would tell my parents. But other than immediate family, I wouldn't say anything.

This was partly driven by fear. I didn't know what the reaction would be to my decision; I worried that it might not be received well and my project would never get off the ground.

But perhaps the biggest reason I didn't tell anyone was that I wanted to see how my journey would impact others—treating it like a science experiment. If I told colleagues or friends about my decision, it might affect the way they communicated with me.

If I didn't respond to a text, would they find another way to get in touch or give up? What better way to find out than by not saying a word?

My strategy was that if someone asked, I would tell them, but otherwise I wouldn't go out of my way to say what I was doing.

We were on vacation in South Carolina the night I turned off my phone for the year. I wrote in my journal that night:

My hope for the next year is that turning off my phone will be a time for me to reconnect. Reconnect with God. Reconnect with my wife. Reconnect with my children. Reconnect with my friends. Reconnect with myself. Signing off. December 31, 9:50 p.m., Isle of Palms, SC.

Withdrawal

I immediately felt withdrawal symptoms when I turned off my phone. Even on vacation, when we should all seek a bit more disconnection than usual, I felt like a part of me was missing.

It was weird to leave the hotel room or drive in the car with nothing to check.

I remember on the first full day of my detox, January 1, 2020, driving to the grocery store at night by myself in an unfamiliar place. Lauren wrote directions for me on a sheet of paper, as well as a shopping list. For almost a decade, I'd relied on GPS technology as my compass. I couldn't remember the last time I drove based on handwritten directions.

It was scary having to navigate turn by turn, even if the store was only ten minutes away, without a comforting automated voice directing me to my destination.

But when I pulled up to the Harris Teeter in Isle of Palms, I felt empowered. Forget that my back and palms were covered in sweat from nerves, it energized me that I could get to a grocery store on my own without a GPS. Ditto with the shopping list.

Usually when I went shopping, I would have an email or text from Lauren with a list of the items I needed to buy. I would text if an item on the list wasn't there, or if I found something that looked appetizing to see if she wanted it.

Food shopping became one big back-and-forth where I would stay glued to my phone. A text exchange would look like:

"Hey Lauren, no blueberry bagels, but I can get everything."

"Are there plain?"

"Let me check. No, no plain. Just cinnamon raisin and everything."

"Okay, let's just skip it."

"Really, no bagels?"

"OK, get some if you want, but not cinnamon raisin."

"OK, will get everything."

"Thanks, love you!"

But with no way to message to discuss purchases, I felt unburdened. I proceeded from one aisle to the next with a sense of freedom that I can only imagine Americans felt when the first grocery store opened up nearly a century ago.

And then came the checkout line. As I stood with several people in front of me, I came to the sudden realization that I had nothing to do. There were no emails or messages to check, no online surfing to be done. There was just me and my cart of groceries.

I was uncomfortable. I decided that I would make myself look busy.

I scanned some of the magazines on the nearby shelf. Most were tabloids, so my perusal didn't last long. Then I looked over the expiration dates of the food in the cart. All fine.

There was nothing else to do. I didn't know what else to do with myself, so I just stared straight ahead, blankly.

I must look like an idiot, I thought to myself.

Then out of nowhere, I started to daydream. I thought about the beach and our plans for the next day. I could feel the cold sand between my toes as I watched the waves crashing. I thought about our three-year-old's smiling face on the playground earlier that morning as we got on the see-saw together. I could hear our seven-month-old's laugh when I put him in his bopper for play time before dinner and see his inquisitive look as he stared at the toy animals dangled in front of him.

I transported to a different place.

After day one of my project, I quickly learned that I would have to embrace silence, to be comfortable enough in my own skin to realize that there would be moments when I would have nothing to do.

I also realized how hyperaware I was of everyone's smartphone use around me.

The Haze Lifts

After a few days at the beach in Charleston, we surprised our oldest and made the six-hour drive south on I-95 to Disney World.

On our first morning, we boarded a crowded bus to Epcot. Cheery Disney songs played on the speakers overhead. Sitting next to us were two grandparents with a high school–aged grandson bobbing his head in between them. At first, I thought he might be enjoying the "Cruella De Vil" song as it played in the background on the bus, but then noticed the AirPods in his ears. His grandparents would speak to him occasionally, not realizing he couldn't hear them.

Up the steps at the other end of the bus, a family of five huddled together. The parents looked to be in their forties, the kids between the ages five and twelve wearing colorful shoes that lit up as they kicked their legs gleefully, each with their own smartphone. It looked like they were playing video games, fervently tapping away on their screens.

In front of us sat two parents and their teenage daughter. All three were wearing Disney shirts and excitedly looking at Disney video clips on their phones, occasionally talking about rides they might go on that day.

Next to them sat a grandmother, parents, and teenage boy. Both parents were glued to their phones, while their son clearly wasn't allowed to have one yet. He looked straight ahead, bored, as if whatever his parents were looking at wasn't interesting.

"Why do we have to wear these wristbands?" the boy asked his mom at one point, breaking out of his dull trance. The question was innocent, sincere.

The mom looked up from her phone. "When you walk around Disney," she explained kindly, "everyone wears a magic band. You wouldn't want to have to take a piece of paper in and out of your bag all day to get on rides, would you?"

The boy shrugged, staring straight ahead again, as his mom looked back down at her phone. It seemed like he was vying for his parents' attention, without much success. I realized that I was that same parent just days prior.

As we waited in line for It's a Small World at Magic Kingdom the next day, a petite, middle-aged woman in front of us was on her Facebook feed, scrolling down quickly, stopping to watch a video every few seconds.

"Mommy, Mommy. I want to be picked up," her five-year-old son started whining.

"Mmm hmm, I hear you honey," she'd say, holding her phone in one hand, keeping her son at arm's length with the other.

"Mommy, pick me up, pick me up."

I couldn't tell what she was streaming, but the boy continued to whine, and the mom continued to ignore him.

The boy eventually got picked up. When he did, he pressed his head against his mom's shoulder, grateful for her embrace. Seconds later, she placed the boy next to her on the seat of a boat. It had been twenty-five minutes since he had first asked to be picked up.

Later that day, as we waited in line for an autograph from Tinker Bell, a brother and sister were getting wild behind us, pushing each other. At one point, the boy fell into my leg. It didn't hurt so I ignored it but felt slightly irked. I looked at the mom, hoping to make eye contact so she'd get control of her kids. She was on her phone though, not paying attention.

A minute later the girl pushed her brother right at me this time, my leg nearly buckling from the contact. "Please stop it!" I snapped. The mom didn't hear me.

Growing up, I always had an image of Disney World being the happiest place on earth. Soaring on the Peter Pan ride or getting spooked in the Haunted Mansion still puts a smile on my face. But as I looked at the throngs of people around the park, so many of them glued to their smartphones, I began to question it all.

A Bright New Reality

After our vacation, it was a return to reality, back to work, school, and our former routines.

But it wasn't totally familiar to me without a smartphone. It was better. I noticed immediate improvements in my focus at work, in relationships, finding time for hobbies, and with investing in myself.

Without my smartphone on at the office, I felt more disciplined. I brought a notepad and pen to meetings, and my information retention improved. When I started to work at home remotely because of the coronavirus pandemic, I told colleagues to call my landline house phone if something came up. So, colleagues knew if there was an emergency there was a way to reach me.

With most communication happening over email and Zoom, I only received one call on my house phone in 2020.

Without being able to text throughout the day, Lauren and I spent time each evening catching each other up on the day's events. I looked forward to these sessions. Without the distraction of a phone, I started setting aside more time for the two of us to spend together. And our relationship grew as a result.

For our boys, I could tell how much they appreciated me not constantly checking my phone. When I took them out for walks or to the pool or playground, they had my undivided attention, which wasn't the case before. I had a newfound appreciation for being a father, something for which I was grateful.

It is important to note that a number of relationships with my friends suffered. I'm fairly sure this was because those relationships were largely based around texting. Without being able to send each other quick messages, we fell out of touch.

But for three of my dearest friends, we grew closer. Because we were forced to call each other, low-effort communication was replaced by high-quality conversation. Instead of sending each other frequent text messages, we set aside time to talk on the phone. Even my wife appreciated this because when my friends called our house phone, she got to catch up with them as well.

With the newfound free time I had each night, I was also able to rekindle past hobbies.

In middle school, I loved to play chess. I remember watching the movie *Searching for Bobby Fischer* and being taken in by the focus and creativity needed to master the game. I never competed in chess tournaments, but I played during lunch with friends, and even started a chess team my freshman year of high school.

Because most of my friends had other interests, however, I gradually stopped playing. During the pandemic, I set aside time each night to play online, challenging friends and colleagues. It became a source of connection during an isolating time.

I also started playing golf more, something that had taken a back seat before 2020. The idea to invest more time in golf came from walks around our neighborhood. As I pushed our one-year-old around in the stroller, I started to daydream about playing. I remember coming back home after one walk and telling Lauren that I wanted to make golf a priority again. It's an undeniably time-consuming game, but with hours freed up by not having a phone it felt more reasonable.

I also began to keep a daily journal. With more time and space to think with my phone off, I wanted to capture ideas and reflections around what I was experiencing.

Then there was the pandemic. When I had planned my yearlong phoneless odyssey, I never could've anticipated that a once-in-a-generation virus would upend our lives. But as isolating as the pandemic was, having my phone off made the experience easier. With so much negative news each day, I found it less stressful to leave the house without seeing the latest headline on CNN.com or receiving an anxiety-provoking text from a family member or friend. We subscribed to one print newspaper, the *Wall Street Journal*, and reading the headlines each day was enough for me.

Cell Phones, by the Numbers

- According to the World Economic Forum, in 2022 there were more than 8.6 billion mobile phone subscriptions in the world. That means there are more mobile devices in the world than people (7.6 billion people as of that date).

- Most mobile phones in use are smartphones. The number of smartphones in the world totals 7.2 billion, and that number continues to grow

- In the United States, 97 percent of people between the ages of 18 and 49 own a smartphone.

The most common uses for smartphones include:

1. Internet searches/web browsing
2. Phone calls
3. Listening to music
4. Using social media apps
5. Sharing/sending photos and videos
6. Banking
7. Shopping
8. Global positioning system/navigation/location-based services
9. Video calls
10. Payment apps

What I Missed

Similar to what I asked Nick Castellanos, you might be wondering whether there were any moments during the year where I got burned by not having a smartphone.

Aside from some minor inconveniences, such as not being able to use GPS or easily log into financial accounts, there were only two specific moments I put in my journal as upsetting for the lack of a smartphone. Both had to do with gathering enough participants for prayer services, known in Judaism as a minyan. On two separate occasions, people messaged me to help ensure a quorum but never got a response. Although it upset me to think that I might have let people down, the reward I felt throughout the year by not having my smartphone outweighed these two negative experiences (which could've been avoided by following the steps in the next chapter).

Eventually, the day arrived. It was December 31, 2020, the last day of my journey, at 11:59 p.m., one minute from being able to turn my phone back on. Lauren was with me in our den, capturing the moment on video. I sat on a black swivel office chair in front of my computer, a wide grin on my face.

I wondered what would happen next. It had been twelve months since I last turned on my phone. Would it have trouble downloading all of the notifications? The new emails, texts, WhatsApp messages, and iPhone software upgrades?

I had received emails throughout the year from people who'd messaged me, gotten no response, and were asking if I was still alive. Would I get more of those? Would a message pop up that I wished I had seen earlier?

I turned on my phone, the signature Apple icon appeared on the opening screen. The icons on the home screen loaded. We waited, anxious to see what would pop up.

After a few minutes, I looked at the screen and realized something weird. Nothing was happening.

"That's strange," I said to Lauren.

I tapped on the Messages icon. Then I opened WhatsApp. All of the most recent messages were from December 31, 2019.

It would take another half hour before I realized that because of the prolonged period I went without using my phone, all of the incoming messages from my detox year likely got lost in the digital ether.

I appreciated the irony. We worry so much about what we'll miss when we turn off our phones, even for a day. I turned off mine for an entire year, and I felt like I hadn't missed a thing.

"What are you going to do now?" Lauren asked me, as amused as I was.

I smiled, then powered the phone down. "It's late, I'm going to get some sleep," I said.

. . . . .

As I began to open up and tell people about my journey, the most common reaction I heard was, "Oh my gosh, I wish I could do that." So many people, I realized, yearned for a way to break free from their phones and live deeper, more meaningful lives.

By the end of this book, you'll have the strategies and tools you need to live a more fulfilling life with or without your smartphone.

But it's important for me to say up front that I will not once make the case that you shouldn't own a smartphone (I still own one!). Nor is this book a diatribe against technology. My livelihood—overseeing website strategy for a top law school—absolutely depends on technology.

Rather, this book is a guide to resetting your relationship with your phone to get back something finite: time.

To begin, you will need to commit to something that will likely make you uncomfortable; the first step is the detox.

CHAPTER 2

The Detox: Turning Off Your Smartphone

Science came naturally to Adam Weiss.

Growing up in Youngstown, Ohio, to parents who owned a laundromat, Weiss attended Ohio State University as a chemistry and neuroscience double major, then entered the PhD chemistry program at University of Chicago in 2018.

Weiss characterized his PhD work as a "high-pressure environment." To pursue an academic career, "you have to do everything you can to get ahead," he told me. "For every person that's working sixty hours a week, there's someone else who's working eighty hours a week."

He had to wear a lot of hats—teaching, grading, pushing his research forward—but he explained to me that he was only doing "the bare minimum."

A major obstacle for Weiss in achieving his goals: his smartphone.

Working in the vaccine lab on campus, Weiss would set up experiments. As the experiments ran, he'd have time to get other things done, including reading academic papers, writing scholarly articles, or reaching out to collaborators.

Instead of furthering his career though, Weiss would spend most of his time on his phone.

"I'd be in my lab and I'd be playing on my phone, whether on Reddit or whatever website instead of actually doing the work that I needed to get done," he said. "I was just not being productive."

But work wasn't the only problem area.

His social life was negatively impacted by his phone. Weiss had a close group of friends in Chicago, but the nature of those friendships was changing, shifting to more digital communication between smartphones.

He'd get memes sent to him throughout the day. His friends started using TikTok. Most of them had iPhones, so they'd often check each other's location, something Weiss described as "invasive."

Then he learned that his friends made a group text message thread without him—and began feeling less connected to them.

Things came to a boil for Weiss in the fall of 2021. Weiss went to an event with his friends in Chicago where they were all mostly looking at their phones instead of interacting with the people around them.

"We're not connecting with each other in the way that we should be connecting," Weiss thought.

Back in his room, still disturbed by the experience, Weiss went on his phone to see how much time he was spending on it each day. When he saw that he was dedicating five hours a day to it, he was alarmed. He started to realize how much of a negative impact his phone was having on his life.

Weiss decided to go to the university mental health services to see a therapist, who drew the same conclusion he already had: His smartphone use was causing too much disruption in his life.

Weiss did some research on alternative phone options and was excited to find one that seemed to fit his needs: a Light Phone, marketed as one "designed to be used as little as possible."

Without an attractive display, web browser, email, social media, or apps, Weiss believed the phone could eliminate many of the distractions that were causing him problems.

He turned off his smartphone and switched his SIM card into the Light Phone. The first week was challenging, as Weiss experienced withdrawal. "I had a headache. I just kept on whipping out this Light Phone and looking for something that just never came," he said.

In the lab, as his experiments were running, and with nothing alluring to reach for, Weiss would sit and feel bored. Seeking to capitalize on the absence of his smartphone, he was determined to do something meaningful with his time.

He started printing papers to read. He wrote a scholarly review about polymers in immunology that got published and cited.

"I just started filling my time with real things instead of fake things," he said. "Doomscrolling never ends, whereas, if you work on a real thing, you get a tangible output at the end . . . if you doomscroll for sixty hours, you've just made it sixty hours down the page."

With several fewer hours per day on his phone he had more space to think, to come up with new ideas. He also became more involved with his PhD program, becoming the director of graduate student initiatives in the chemistry department.

At first, Weiss's friends thought he was crazy for simplifying his phone. But over time they accepted that if they needed to reach him, they would have to call.

"The memes that I was getting twenty times a day over text message were not having any positive impact whatsoever on my life," Weiss explained. "What mattered was when we go to hang out, we go get a drink after work, being there together with people, that's what mattered at the end of the day."

Turning off his smartphone and switching to the Light Phone achieved exactly what Weiss was looking for: a reset. He spent two months using the Light Phone and began to evaluate the change he'd made. He decided he was grateful to have gotten away from his smartphone and was happy with the results he achieved, but he didn't like the Light Phone's interface.

He switched to a Cat S22 Flip, which offered more functionality than the Light Phone, but was enough of a pain to use that it wasn't a distraction. It had a T9 (text on nine keys) keyboard, which added enough friction to discourage Weiss from responding to messages right away.

Like me, Weiss never got rid of his smartphone—he'll turn it on for cross-country trips or if he's going to a concert and needs it for e-ticketing. He just switches over the SIM card from his Cat to his iPhone.

He said he uses his Cat 80 percent of the time, and his smartphone the other 20 percent of the time, a balance that he prefers. When he's not using his smartphone, he leaves it off and doesn't take it with him. "I don't have the self-control," he told me.

Two months away from his smartphone gave Weiss the balance and perspective he needed. He now averages 45 to 60 minutes a day on his phone, an 85 percent decrease from before.

Looking back on his detox experience, he said he not only won back time each day, but also regained autonomy in his life.

"It felt like I wasn't living up to my potential," Weiss told me. "I needed to find a system that works."

. . . . .

Dopamine is most commonly associated with reward and pleasure. By switching off your phone, you help prime your brain to embrace new behaviors, leading to an increase in dopamine from more productive activities.

"Even if your long-term goal is moderation, you should start with a period of abstinence as a way to reset reward pathways," explains Dr. Anna Lembke, author of *Dopamine Nation* and a Stanford University professor of psychiatry who specializes in addiction.

The first thing to understand is that turning your smartphone off will not be easy. The second is that you don't want to embark on this process haphazardly. You will need to prepare.

WHY HACKS DON'T WORK

For most people, the smartphone is such a pervasive tool that simple "hacks" won't make a big enough difference. Referred to as *harm reduction* in psychological terms, hacks are ubiquitous in newspaper articles and other self-help books. That's why so many of us are trying them.

"They're based in good ideas," said Dr. Ed Spector, a therapist in Maryland who specializes in digital addiction. "But all of these sexy little self-help things aren't really based in research." As Spector explained, most of us are just "winging it" when we try hacks or small changes in our smartphone use.

"Hacks tend in my experience to never be enough by themselves," said screen addiction specialist Dr. Clifford Sussman. "And at best and at worst, they tend to always fail."

Many of the mental health experts I consulted told me that taking the path of moderation involves so much effort to not slip that in most cases it isn't worth it. It's easier and more worthwhile to find a better way of functioning.

Over the course of four years and countless interviews researching this book, I can say with confidence that the allure of the phone is too strong to simply hack.

Below are some of the most common hacks people try and why they don't work:

- **Deleting Social Media:** This is perhaps the most common hack people try to address their smartphone use. The problem with it is that even if you delete an app such as Instagram or X, you'll still have all of the other addictive parts of your phone to explore. This includes messaging, internet browsing, video and music streaming, and gaming, among others.

- **A Digital Sabbath:** This involves picking a day of the week to turn off your phone. It's a great idea in principle, but as I learned all too well (see page 20), once you're using your smartphone again after twenty-four hours, the compulsive need to check it throughout the day will quickly return. I compared it earlier to telling someone who is a cigarette addict not to smoke for one day a week. They might be successful for that one day, but once the twenty-four hours passes, that person will be right back to smoking again.

- **A Rubber Band:** Put a rubber band around your phone. The idea behind it is that when you reach for your phone, it creates an obstacle to using it. The sight of the rubber band can also provide a reminder to think twice before using your device. Unfortunately, unless the phone is locked and you don't have the key, you'll still find a way to use your phone, even with a rubber band.

- **The Phone Foyer Method:** Coined by Cal Newport, the definition for this approach is as follows:

When you get home after work, you put your phone on a table in your foyer near your front door. Then—and this is the important part—you leave it there until you next leave the house.

In addition to my own experience, I heard mixed results about this approach. Although it is beneficial to have to walk to a specific place of the house to check for updates—ensuring you don't bring it into the bedroom or kitchen—you will feel a constant pull to want to check it when you are home. It also doesn't address what happens when you leave the house.

- **Airplane Mode:** Putting your phone in airplane mode helps make you *feel* like you're offline, but knowing that your phone is only a swipe away from being back in full addictive mode can make this strategy challenging to maintain. Even in airplane mode, you will likely still find yourself tapping your phone to view photos, play games, and check for messages—even if you know nothing new is going to come in.

- **Grayscale:** Setting your phone to black-and-white can make the phone less visually appealing. But according to a 2023 study, setting your phone to grayscale may reduce the amount of time you spend on your phone, but won't change how often you compulsively check it.

That is why we need to do something comprehensive: a reset. That's where the detox comes in, and the first step is to turn off your smartphone.

Preparation

Preparation is essential if you want your detox to be a success.

In the interviews I conducted, most people took at least one month to think about how the detox would impact others personally and professionally.

"Because these devices are so integrated into our everyday lives, including our professional and family lives, it's really important to anticipate and prepare for the quit date," Lembke told me.

Ensure that those closest to you—your parents, children, dear friends, and colleagues—are supporting you in this endeavor.

Don't be afraid to speak up.
Make the case for why quitting is important to you.

Dr. Hilarie Cash, chief clinical officer of reSTART Life, a treatment center in Bellevue, Washington, for people suffering from screen addiction, argues that having a good support system in place is critical to make a behavior change of this magnitude.

"If you are trying to do it all on your own, it can be very, very difficult and often not successful," she said.

Speak to loved ones about what you are about to do.

Be open with your employer if you feel that turning off your smartphone could have an impact on your work.

A conversation with your boss could go something like this: "I just read a book by Richard Simon called *Unplug*. I'm really unhappy with how I use my smartphone. Simon recommends turning it off as a good first step to reset the relationship. I will still be reachable by Zoom or email. This is very important to me. Will you support me in doing this?"

When it's a question of mental health and optimizing your life, you'd be surprised at how open and supportive people are.

Take your time during the preparation process, don't rush it.

"You can't just detox quickly," said Dr. Ed Spector. "If you detox quickly without preparing yourself for it, it is going to be really problematic."

Spector recalled one client who was detoxing from a gaming addiction. During the detox, his client called from the platform of a train station, ready to jump on the tracks. Spector was able to calm him from doing anything drastic, but what his client said was chilling.

He said, "Doc, I have hours a week that I didn't have before. I have no interests. No hobbies. Never kissed a girl. Don't have a driver's license. I'm twenty years old. What the fuck am I supposed to do?"

Spector emphasized to me that anyone preparing for a detox needs to first evaluate what they want to achieve—and that includes determining what your replacement behaviors will be.

HOW TO PITCH THE DETOX TO PARTNERS, FAMILY, AND FRIENDS

When you are ready to reset the relationship with your smartphone, it is important to understand that your decision will have an impact on other people, especially those relationships you hold dearest.

It is also important to not keep the reset a secret: Establishing a support group is critical.

That's why you should talk openly with your partner, family, and close friends when you are ready to break up with your phone.

For the conversation with your "inner circle," here are my recommendations:

- **Emphasize mutual gain:** Don't make it about you. Approach the topic from a position of mutual gain, especially with a spouse or partner. The argument for breaking up with your phone should be "about us." It isn't like you are asking to play golf for five hours every Sunday, as well as going to the driving range three days a week. Present it as a value add for everyone. In the short term, it will likely be difficult. But from the case studies in this book, you'll find that once you get to the other side, everyone will be better off.

- **Show compassion:** Present your argument with sincerity and affection. Believe in what you are saying and speak with conviction.

- **Establish an emergency valve:** This is often the biggest concern with a phone breakup. It might be difficult on someone else that you won't be as available as you were before.

Although an emergency is unlikely, put systems in place so that you can be reached if one occurs. Alternative communication methods you might suggest include email, work phone, landline, or the classic, knock on my front door. (See page 144 for more.)

- **Ask for support:** If you just tell someone you are doing a detox, they might think to themselves, *Why are you telling me this?* Make sure your conversation includes a request for support.

- **Paint a picture:** Explain how you are going to fill your time without your smartphone and give real-life examples. This could involve reinvesting in work or relationships, or pursuing a hobby. Be specific.

- **Relate success stories:** This is not a marketing ploy, but mention that you read this book. Especially if no one close to you is familiar with this process, it will add legitimacy if you cite the strategies and/or profiles that you think will resonate.

Evaluation

Before a detox, Spector tells clients to **take a blank sheet of paper and create columns at the top of the page with a category listed atop each for what matters to you in life.**

Sample categories could include intellectual, spiritual, athletic, community, social, charity, and personal investment. Once you've identified the most important values in your life, write in activities that fit within those categories. For example, if you want to join a soccer league, add that to an athletic or community column. If you want to attend church twice a week, add it to spiritual, community, or personal investment.

Here's an example of what your sheet of paper could look like.

Community	Social	Personal Investment
• Sign up for the open play pickleball league near my house. • Attend church every Sunday morning with group Bible study. • Join the Thriller book club that my brother is a part of.	• Go out to dinner one night a week with a friend. • Write a handwritten love note to my spouse or partner once a week. • Call my parents every Sunday night.	• 45 minutes on the elliptical each evening, except Fridays. • Read one chapter a day. • Spend 10 minutes every morning for contemplation and reflection. • Write in my journal before sleep.

Once your sheet is complete, step away from it for a week, then come back to it and refine it further. Once it's complete, you have your menu. When you start your detox and find yourself with hours of extra free time, you can check your sheet of paper and simply decide what you want to order.

If you want to increase your chances for success, make a copy and share the sheet with at least one person you are close with, and schedule check-ins to ensure you are following through.

The advantage of setting up priorities for yourself is that if you step away from your smartphone and don't have a way to fill your time, you could experience not only greater withdrawal but also psychological harm.

But here's my caveat and suggestion: **Try to make it so that the categories you include aren't screen dependent.**

There may be exceptions of course. If you're setting out to learn a new language, for example, getting a virtual tutor could be helpful. But try your best to commit to activities that don't involve screens.

The reason, as we'll explore later, is that with the loss of your smartphone, your mind will crave high-dopamine activities as a replacement, such as using a computer.

If you have a plan that includes high-quality replacement goals and activities, "you just shine," Spector told me.

Optimize Your Home Environment

Setting up the proper home environment is essential when doing your detox.

Dr. Clifford Sussman told me that during the pandemic, when many of his clients shifted to online classes on their computers, they were forced to learn at home on the same screen that they were using to play games like *Fortnite*.

"I likened it to drinking water in a bar," he said. "Good luck with that, especially if you have a history of alcoholism."

Sussman works with clients on changing the home environment so that specific rooms are for high-dopamine activities with screens, while other spaces are for low-dopamine activities.

This means that screens don't belong in the bedroom, which signals to your brain that it's a place for sleep. They also shouldn't be in your dining room or kitchen, signaling that it's time to eat. Ditto the den, which should signal to you that it's for low-dopamine activities requiring more patience and effort, such as reading. If there's a specific room or corner of your home for screens, when you leave that space, the devices stay there. That way, if you wanted to sneak into the room to get a "quick hit," there is a delay—you can't get it instantly.

Keeping one place in the house for high-dopamine activities like the computer and television, and ensuring that it's at least a little separate from the rest of the house, will help your detox and beyond.

Most of of the writing for this book was done on my deck in the winter of 2024. I wore a winter coat and beanie with my computer set on a table or folding chair. If I wrote inside the house, I would have been surrounded by distractions. So the deck became my writing space.

Duration

How long you do a smartphone detox varies, but after speaking to experts and interviewing people who went through the experience, **I strongly recommend turning off your smartphone for at least two months.**

There are plenty of articles that recommend thirty days. But, as I learned firsthand, it can take several weeks just to get past the feelings of withdrawal after you turn off your smartphone. I was nervous when I didn't have something to reach for and had nothing to do. I had to get comfortable being present—and that took time.

Dr. Hilarie Cash describes this withdrawal period as a time when "the brain is up regulating again to normal function. And people don't feel very happy during that time."

"That first month is basically your brain coming back to normal," she added.

Of all the people I interviewed, the shortest duration I heard for a successful detox was two months. From there, the range varied from two months to one year to four years to permanently.

"There's no doubt that the longer people go the better that they feel and the more that they begin to develop other habits, other ways of being present," said Dr. Anna Lembke.

Withdrawal

The feelings of withdrawal you have when you turn off your smartphone can be mild and last only a few days. But for some, they can be severe.

"I really put a strong emphasis on mindful awareness of withdrawal and how hard that can be and how withdrawal from digital devices can be physical," Lembke explained.

Physical symptoms might include stomachaches, headaches, sweating, and panic attacks. Young adults and children going through a detox may have meltdowns or look completely dysregulated.

But after a few weeks pass and you get past the feelings of withdrawal, you will get something back: time.

And that's when you will begin to have a clearer vision.

Reintegration

Among the dozens of people I interviewed, most decided that they did not want to bring a smartphone back into their lives.

But for those who do, it can often be challenging.

Dr. Marc Potenza is a professor of psychiatry at the Yale School of Medicine who specializes in addiction and impulse control disorders. He said there are biological changes when people with gambling or alcohol addictions reintroduce the behavior to their lives, either with a sip of alcohol or a visit to the casino. Smartphones have yet to be investigated in the same manner, but Potenza encourages people to be cautious.

"In some ways, it may be playing with fire," he told me. "You may not get burned—you may feel the warmth—but you may also get burned."

If you do decide to bring a smartphone back into your life (which we'll review in chapter 5), planning for that period is as important as preparing to detox—proper guardrails are needed to make it a success.

CHAPTER 3

Breakup Styles

Thankfully, there are a number of different ways to break up with your phone. And while all involve some kind of detox, there is flexibility to choose one that best fits your life and needs. In this chapter, I'll present four detox approaches that emerged from my research and the extensive interviews with those who've tried—and succeeded—with each. Their stories, as well as concrete tips to help you, are included here.

Whether you are a physician, lawyer, marketer, or educator, I'm confident you'll find a breakup style to work for you.

Let's begin with the first and most common approach.

Option 1: Simplify Your Phone

For years, Seth Lavin prided himself on being available to anyone who wanted to speak with him—no matter the time of day.

With more than 700 students and 100 staff under his watch, Lavin is the principal of Brentano Math & Science Academy, a pre-K–8th-grade public school on the northwest side of Chicago.

In addition to his core responsibility of educating some of Chicago's youngest minds, Lavin spent hours every day communicating with teachers, families, and students on a wide range of issues, with many conversations kicking off by text message.

Most days, Lavin found himself engaged in more than 100 text conversations, with at least 15 individual texts embedded within each thread. He tried to be disciplined and not send text messages after work hours, but found that colleagues had issues surface during the school day that they wanted to resolve before the next day. As a result, there was little separation between Lavin's workday and evening time. It all blended together.

At home, when Lavin wasn't sending messages he would look for a quick escape from the busyness of the day, often by mindlessly surfing the internet and perusing social media on his phone.

Eventually, Lavin began to realize how out of control his habits were and decided to check how much time he was spending on his iPhone each day. Six hours.

Six hours might surprise you, or not. But if you add the number up across an entire calendar year, it's ninety-one days. Or three months on his phone.

As difficult as accepting that number was, Lavin told me that what hurt most about his phone use was seeing how much it affected his kids.

"Ultimately, they were noticing that I was on this phone all the time and it was having a negative impact on their lives. And I think that's what made me feel really bad," he lamented.

Both of his kids attend Brentano—and they associated his phone with his job. One day, Lavin's kids told him, "You know, you should get a different job. Like you should get a job where you don't need your phone."

One of them added, "Do you think you have to be the principal of our school to take care of us? Because we'd be okay."

Lavin was floored. "It is an incredible thing for them to say as they are processing, that maybe our dad is doing this job out of some sense of duty and we should release him of that. They were doing a lot of work to sort of absolve me of it," he explained.

As Lavin reflected more on his relationship with his kids, he was able to pinpoint one specific personal choice that allowed him to be present.

Whenever Lavin took his kids out for activities, such as the zoo, he would leave his phone in the car.

"Some of the most special times for me in their childhood are times that I had my phone in the car, and they were special [times] because I was there," he said.

Lavin wanted to experience that feeling he had when he took his kids out for special activities, but all the time. He began contemplating what life would be like if he didn't have a smartphone and how it would impact his career, his wife, and his kids.

Making the Switch

In the summer of 2023, the Lavins hosted friends: a couple with two kids who were close in age to theirs. Both of the parents had basic phones.

"I think that was a point that made this thing that I was thinking about feel more possible," said Lavin.

Over the next few months, Lavin researched basic phone options and decided to buy a Kyocera flip phone. He transferred the SIM card from his iPhone to it.

When he made the switch, he told me that he felt "totally giddy."

"I felt just like a total ecstatic thrill of like, 'I'm released. I'm free.'"

There were some aspects of the smartphone Lavin missed, including easy access to music, GPS, Uber, and the camera.

But when I connected with Lavin several months after he made the switch, he told me that the immediate gains he experienced far outweighed the instant availability of music and maps.

"I am spending more time with my kids and wife," he told me. "I notice those relationships deepening and that feels really good."

He told me that his ten-year-old started doing a one-mile run on the treadmill in their basement every day. His son asked Lavin to sit with him while he runs so that he has company.

Before switching to the basic phone, Lavin was convinced he would have sat next to the treadmill and spent most of the time on his smartphone. Now they talk—a daily conversation they wouldn't have had if he was responding to messages or checking emails.

As both a parent and a principal, Lavin firmly believes that kids need "space to fill up," and smartphones are a clear obstacle.

"You just have to be there, ready for them. Because when they want to talk or share or think or ask, you're not in control of that. But if it happens and you're not there, if you miss it, if you're looking away, if you're not listening, if they call your name and you don't answer, you miss it and so do they . . . I noticed that my son will turn to me and tell me this thing happened at school, or 'my friend said this,' it's like those things happen on their schedule, these moments of connecting that they're looking for. And so the difference is to be ready for these moments when they're seeking connection. And I think when I had the smartphone, it's all on my terms, it's like I'm mostly not here."

Lavin admits that he still uses his basic phone more than he'd like, but because of the hassle that comes with using it, it also sets up barriers. "It's not that it's clunky, it's just not that good. If I'm receiving too many text messages at once, it can't handle it. It puts up a message, basically an error message that says that this phone is trying to do too many things. And so that slows me down," he said.

I asked Lavin what the response has been from teachers and families now that he takes longer to respond to messages.

"I'm sure if you're somebody waiting for me to write back to you, and I'm not, you wish I had a smartphone so I could write back sooner, but I don't actually think that makes the school that I lead worse. And there are some ways in which being slightly less reactive makes things better," he told me.

Lavin believes we've started to overcommunicate in schools and in a lot of workplaces. He sees this as a danger, that we might be communicating so much that we're talking more about work than actually doing it.

In line with his own personal thinking, Lavin took the step of banning phones from school in the fall of 2023, equipping classrooms with lockboxes that the kids call "cell phone prisons."

Lavin told me the policy isn't perfect and that some kids will put a fake phone in the lockbox and then be equipped with a second phone to keep in a pocket, but the importance of having a place where the phone is kept away has made for a better school experience.

Being a principal for the last ten years, Lavin has seen firsthand what smartphones have done to children at the school.

"You can tell when a kid in class takes out their phone because they just disappear. Like they just stop being there. And you can tell when kids get their phones because kids who suddenly own a phone, their personalities change," he said.

When Lavin switched the SIM card over to his basic phone, he didn't get rid of his smartphone. He still turns it on from time to time to make financial transactions. And when he does, he's blown away by how incredible and brilliant the device is.

"It's too much to have and to hold and to exist and to try and restrain yourself with," he said.

Like so many of us, Lavin describes himself as being easily distracted. His mind shifts quickly to different topics, and that can make it difficult for him to be in the moment with nothing to do.

"It's not like sitting there with my thoughts is easy," he said. "But I like that person a lot better than the person who's on their phone for six hours a day."

QUIT TIP 2 Make These Two Investments

Purchasing this book was an investment for your detox, for which I am grateful, but I am going to recommend that you consider making two additional investments.

The first is a camera.

When Anthony Donataccio and Michele Perry turned off their smartphones (see page 121), they bought a small, portable camera that captures high-quality photos and videos.

"It's just using a camera that's not connected to anything . . . and for me it's just really cool because I am so much more present," said Donataccio.

He and Perry recall that when they used to travel with their smartphones, they would spend time posting their photos to Instagram, figuring out what captions they would write and which hashtags to use, a process that would sometimes take half an hour and leave them feeling on edge.

Using a standalone camera, Donataccio downloads his photos onto his computer and backs them up to the cloud, then emails them to family directly rather than posting on social media.

"I actually get to capture little things that are really cool and enjoy the experience a lot more," he told me.

For Kate Emmons (see page 79), to eliminate the distraction that comes with taking photos on a phone and the inevitable context shifting, she purchased two Canon cameras.

"I find that there is a sweetness to be found in the process of taking photos, then coming home and loading them into my computer to view and edit however [many] I feel drawn to. It's like playtime. . . . I've kind of let this become a process of self-discovery, just like with any other art form," she wrote to me.

Next, I recommend subscribing to a physical newspaper.

Print subscriptions have been on the decline for years, but there are still some quality newspapers available. Rather than endlessly scrolling to get your news, set aside at least twenty minutes each day to read news from a print newspaper, then do your best to not check news sites throughout the day.

As a former journalist, I used to look at news on my phone around the clock. But now that I've taken a step back I can say with conviction that unless you're working at the State Department there is no need for you to be checking news throughout the day. News networks benefit from your incessant scrolling—sadly, you do not.

You will feel less anxious and just as informed if you only read your news once a day. Regardless of where you stand politically, consider subscribing to a newspaper like the *New York Times*, *Wall Street Journal*, or *Washington Post*, and cut out reading online news. Make hard-copy reading a ritual: Read your paper at a specific time, in a specific place. If you commute, read it on the train or bus. Turning each page is more fulfilling than the Russian roulette of swiping, unsure what the algorithm will deliver next.

Although these two investments may seem trivial, it's important to understand that these purchases are telling your brain you are serious about the detox. Putting money behind the effort is a signal that you're invested financially *and* emotionally.

When I wanted to cut sugar out of my diet in 2023, I started to buy $8/box sugar-free cereal. It pained me each time I bought the cereal, but it was a signal to my brain that I better not eat sugary foods or else I had just wasted that money.

If you want your detox to stick, invest in the process.

It's Never Too Early to Quit

Third grade. That may seem like an early age to get a smartphone, but for Josh Haskell it wasn't out of the ordinary.

Most of his peers had one and were on Snapchat and other social media platforms, with many playing mobile games like *Plants vs. Zombies*. The Grand Rapids, Michigan, elementary schooler wasn't at an age for self-reflection, though. He wasn't thinking about screen time—he was living in a digital world like everyone else, spending hours a day on his phone. For Haskell, it all seemed so normal.

But when he reached high school, Haskell started to think about all the time he was wasting. It turned out he was averaging at least three hours a day on his phone, so he made the decision to cut down on screen time.

He tried a number of different ways to make the phone less addictive. He deleted social media applications. He changed the color of his smartphone screen to black-and-white to make it less attractive. He set screen time restrictions. He put his phone on airplane mode.

He tried these approaches for several years as he finished high school and got through his first year and a half at Notre Dame University. And though Haskell cut down his screen time, it still wasn't enough for him.

"The hacks could only take me so far," he told me. "Even if I'm not using the phone, I'm thinking about it in my pocket, or I'm thinking about who texted me or what to say in the group chat. And it goes on and on."

Haskell noticed that whenever he would feel burned-out from schoolwork or feel lonely, he would spend time on his phone.

He finally came to a realization.

"I'll never get to where I want to be unless I just remove the temptation altogether," he said.

In 2022, during Haskell's sophomore year winter break, he drove to a Target store and purchased an Alcatel flip phone, which he could easily swap his smartphone SIM card to.

After he made the switch, Haskell was shocked at the ease of his transition.

"I loved it so much, like right away. I know for a lot of people, it might be hard at first, which is understandable, but for me it was just so freeing," he said. "I was just so present in a way that I had never been before."

The first area of his life that improved was his schoolwork.

Haskell felt he was able to focus in lectures for the entire class without straining himself. When he used to go the library for studying, he would put his smartphone in his backpack. This would create a constant mental battle in his head of whether or not to check his phone, which would drain him. When Haskell made the switch, the mental gymnastics went away.

"The fight doesn't exist because I just hate my phone," he told me.

Haskell's grades improved, and during his senior year, he found out that he was a valedictorian candidate for the 2024 graduating class, one of twenty students who receive the honor each year.

With more time on his hands outside of his academic work, Haskell said that he learned how to play the guitar, started writing poetry, and discovered a love for reading. Before switching to a basic phone, he read one to three school-related books a year. Between his sophomore and senior years, Haskell read fifty, most for pleasure.

Haskell also found time for something that was missing in his life: prayer. As a practicing Catholic who now had more free time, Haskell started going each morning to the chapel in his dorm for twenty-five minutes and then to mass in the afternoon at the basilica.

As impressive as all of these things were, what stood out to me most was how Haskell navigated his social life at college without a smartphone and social media. He said many people in college think that if you delete iMessage, Snapchat, or Instagram, your social life will die. But Haskell said the opposite happened.

"I was being more social than ever in my life," he said.

Because he had a basic phone, Haskell said most people adjusted to not reaching out to him on social media and would call more often, knowing that texting for Haskell had become a hassle.

"Not only did I have more time for friends . . . I also had way more social energy because I wasn't wasting that craving online. So, I had a lot more eagerness to just get out and be social."

Haskell began to view relationships with a fresh perspective. Without being able to look someone up using social media, he told me he approached each first encounter with someone without a shred of bias. He began to discover people for who they really are, versus painting an incomplete picture of someone from their social media account.

Haskell remembers having a difficult conversation with a girlfriend, a relationship he knew deep down wasn't going to work. When he arrived back at his dorm room, he had to figure out what he was going to do.

In the past, he might have taken out his smartphone and started to scroll. Instead, he walked into his room and sat down on his futon. There was nothing to turn on, so he stared. He stared at the wall in front of him.

"You can only stare at a wall for like five or ten minutes before you're like, 'Okay, I need to think about something to do here,'" he said. "And the natural result is I walk over across the hallway and actually hang out with my friends. And that's a harder thing to do than going on my phone, but so much more healthy. And it's actually so good for relationships, that vulnerability to being forced to do that and let people see you be weak versus just the Tylenol of the phone medicating the symptoms without getting to the root."

Haskell wrote a letter to the *Observer*, Notre Dame's student newspaper, about his switch to a basic phone. It would become one of the most-read articles of the year, and friends of Haskell's started to try out basic phones as well.

"My first girlfriend ever actually was because of the article, she emailed me after . . . and then we just started dating. So, it was kind of funny. I kind of thought girls would think it was weird, but it was the opposite," he said.

Switching to a basic phone changed Haskell's perspective on relationships. With less texting and no social media presence, he started to realize who his real friends were. With so many large text message threads and group chats, Haskell found that if you try and be there for everyone, it will be difficult to have authentic relationships.

"It's okay to lose touch with people," he said.

After graduating from college in 2024, Haskell

started a nonprofit that came about from his experience of living a more intentional life with a basic phone.

Haskell, like so many young men, watched pornography online, and the phone made it that much easier to consume. (In November 2022, the fourth most popular website on the Internet was PornHub. With billions of site visits every month, 97% come from mobile devices.)

After switching to a basic phone and being more connected with his faith and aware of his screen time, he started accountability groups on campus for porn consumption. He expected a small group to come forward because of the sensitivity surrounding the topic, but 150 male students showed up.

Based on the success of the pilot at Notre Dame, Haskell's nonprofit, Ethos National, facilitates support and accountability groups on campuses around the country to wean people off of pornography.

"I've been really shocked at how many people have been willing to take leadership roles in this, because (the topic) is so taboo," he said.

Looking back on his life and career trajectory, Haskell sees his decision of switching to a basic phone as a transformative moment.

"The only way you are going to satisfy the desires that lead you to your smartphone is by getting rid of it," he said. "So, try it for a little bit. You can get these things [basic phones] for so cheap. And if you hate it (a basic phone), you hate it. But no one really does."

GUIDELINES FOR SIMPLIFYING YOUR PHONE

Of the dozens of interviews I conducted, the most common detox strategy I found was turning off your smartphone and switching to a basic phone.

Although a 2024 report from Pew indicates that 90 percent of people in the United States use smartphones, there's growing evidence that more people are seeking a simpler alternative.

In a 2023 *Wall Street Journal* story, reporter Kate Morgan found that basic phones were experiencing a renaissance among Gen Z, allowing adolescents to detach from constant notifications.

Nokia reports that it sells tens of thousands of flip phones each month in the United States.

There are many basic phone options, ranging from the most basic like the Light Phone and Gabb, to more sophisticated ones like the Cat S22 Flip or Kyocera DuraXV Extreme+ that host some apps.

I recommend making the basic phone you choose as simple as possible to ensure your detox is a success. Remember: This isn't supposed to be a cakewalk—you will likely feel discomfort switching to a basic phone.

The Light Phone, Alcatel, TCL, Nokia, and Gabb phones are strong contenders in this regard. You can buy an Alcatel flip phone for less than $100 that will give you calling and texting, and that's about it. It technically has an internet browser, but it's hard to use. The T9 (text on nine keys) texting interface requires you to key in each letter, which can be frustrating. Its interface is so unappealing that you won't want to use it very much—and that's the point.

The Light Phone costs several hundred dollars and doesn't have internet or email functionality. The interface uses an e-ink display similar to the Kindle's and is intentionally bland.

After your detox is complete, if you want to continue using a basic phone but with more features, consider the Cat or Kyocera.

By switching the SIM card from your smartphone to your basic phone, you can keep the same phone number and mobile provider.

Below are the seven models of basic phones that came up consistently in the interviews I conducted.

	INTERNET BROWSER	EMAIL	PRICE	TOUCH-SCREEN	GPS	NETWORK	SPOTIFY	PODCASTS
Light Phone	No	No	$299	Yes	Yes	AT&T, Verizon, T-Mobile	No[†]	Yes
Alcatel Go Flip 4	Yes	Yes	$90	No	Yes	T-Mobile (Other Alcatel models are supported by AT&T and Verizon)	No[†]	Yes
Kyocera DuraXV/XA Extreme+	Yes	Yes	$250	No	Yes*	AT&T, Verizon, T-Mobile	Yes*	Yes
Cat S22 Flip	Yes	Yes	$61	Yes	Yes	T-Mobile	Yes	Yes
Nokia 2780	Yes	Yes	$90	No	Yes	AT&T, Verizon, T-Mobile	No[†]	Yes
Gabb	No	No	$150	Yes	Yes[††]	N/A, Gabb has its own plan	No[†]	No
TCL Flip 2	Yes	Yes	$20	No	Yes	Verizon, T-Mobile	Yes*	No

* difficult to install
[†] supports music
[††] filtered

Option 2: Off-by-Default

The South Kaibab Trail is known for its wondrous, 360-degree views of Grand Canyon National Park. The steep, difficult hike leads visitors from all over the world below the rim of the canyon. Because there are few opportunities for shade, it can be an incredibly rewarding yet grueling trip, with temperatures reaching well over 100 degrees Fahrenheit.

For twenty-four-year-old Kate Emmons, the hike was an opportunity to unplug.

A fiction writer from Vermont, Emmons was an avid smartphone user. Aspiring to build a readership online, she had started spending more time on social media apps including Instagram and Facebook. She found herself regularly drawn to her phone throughout the day as notifications popped up, or she'd feel compelled to check how her posts were performing.

As more people began interacting with her over email and social media, Emmons began to recognize a change in how she thought of herself.

"After a while I started noticing, I'm really paying an enormous amount of attention to the interaction I'm getting on these posts," she told me. "And just comparing yourself to others and starting to value yourself based on this content you're creating to share online. I was just so drawn into that every single day."

Because of how distracted she was by her phone, she found that she was becoming less productive with her writing, not reaching the level of focus she was hoping for. It went deeper: Her phone wasn't just impacting her professional career—it was also impacting the relationships she held dearest.

When Emmons and her husband, Tyler, would finish dinner, she'd pick up her smartphone. When she'd look up, Tyler would also be on his phone. This bothered her. She felt like they were together, but not.

So, when Emmons went on a cross-country trip in 2019 with her dad to hike the Grand Canyon in Arizona, she decided to try something new. Researching the trip beforehand, Emmons read that there was no cell phone service below the rim of the canyon. She decided to not take her phone with her on the hike.

After just a few hours in the warm air, she experienced "an awakening."

"I felt better than I had in years," she told me. "I felt so much lighter, so much happier, so much more present in my body in the space I was in . . . I was observing where I was, and what I was doing, and what I was eating, and the sounds I was hearing around me, without any urge or need to share them, because that device to facilitate it was gone. . . . It was this euphoric feeling, and I loved it."

Emmons and her father stayed overnight at a ranch in the canyon. As a severe thunderstorm raged above them, she reflected on the rarity of having no access to technology. She couldn't check email to engage with readers, there were no text messages to see, and she had no social media feeds to refresh. She didn't even know what time it was.

She felt present, her attention undivided.

"I need to figure out how I can have this in my life all the time," she thought.

Immediately after the trip ended, Emmons decided to do something bold—she would turn off her smartphone.

Over the next month, Emmons began planning for the transition. As an author, she still wanted to be able to communicate with her readers and stay in touch with friends. She wondered how she could do both without having her phone on.

She figured out that she could do many of the same things she did on her phone, but on a laptop. And Emmons didn't want to stop using social media, so she decided to focus on only one social media channel, YouTube.

Rather than check her social feeds throughout the day like she did before, she decided that she would set aside time two days a week to produce high-quality videos to improve the lives of fellow writers. Emmons felt that blocking out specific time during the week would be a better recipe than checking her phone throughout the day or more frequent social media posting. She chose quality over quantity.

For family and friends, she gave specific yet simple instructions: If something comes up, call me on my landline at home or send me an email. Emmons's husband, Tyler, was supportive and understanding of her decision to pursue a more fulfilling, focused life without a smartphone.

After two months of deliberative thought and planning, Emmons decided the time was right to begin her detox. She turned off her phone but didn't throw it away, opting to hold on to it. For now.

Making It Permanent

Emmons admitted to having some anxiety about her career and how she was going to publicize her work. But then, because she grew up without a smartphone and didn't get one until late in high school, turning it off felt like "coming home."

The benefits were immediate, she explained.

"My work got a lot better because I was focusing much more on writing, not being interrupted by my phone."

As she devoted her attention to YouTube only, her channel grew, reaching more than thirty thousand subscribers.

"It made it so much less about using social media to build something for myself," she said, "and so much more about how I can help others who are just people on the other side of the screen."

Outside of work, Tyler noticed how much she was growing. "He's like, 'Wow, you're so much happier now,'" she said. "'You're so much more relaxed.'"

Emmons recounted a camping trip she took with Tyler in the Adirondacks, where they made sure there were no distractions. They sat by a fire and told each other stories from when they were kids, reliving old memories. They explored ideas around what they wanted to do in the future, and shared their latest aspirations.

"Wow," she thought to herself, "I'm learning new things about this human being that I've been married to for six years . . ."

She also became closer with her sister, launching a podcast with her called *The Kate and Abbie Show*. Turning off her phone removed what Emmons described as a "third person in the mix," allowing her to be fully present when she was hanging out with her sister or working on their podcast.

"It made me so much more grateful for the conversations and time that I get to have with her," she said.

After Emmons cemented her new habit, she decided it was better to leave her smartphone powered off as its default state. It's a philosophy that I practice as well, something I named *off-by-default*.

The definition for this philosophy is:

The default position of the smartphone should be off. The only time it should be turned on is to accomplish a critical task. After the task is executed, the phone is turned back off.

If there's an emergency or if she wants to check for important texts, Emmons will turn her smartphone on. Otherwise, it remains off.

That means Emmons only turns her phone on once every month to two months.

. . . . .

In 2023, four years after her phone breakup, Emmons decided to stop using her smartphone altogether. She called up her local AT&T store and found the one basic phone in stock, a TCL Flip.

She only uses the phone to make calls when she is traveling, and described the lifestyle change as "refreshing."

When I last connected with her in 2024, she told me that she had just become a registered yoga teacher, a process that took 200 hours of training.

She credits turning off her phone years earlier as a critical piece that gave her the energy to pursue the certification.

"It really amazes me just how *much* we can discover about ourselves when we make conscious choices to quiet our minds and reclaim our own personal power. It's truly a form of self-care," she said.

Model the Right Behavior for Loved Ones

Deirdre Folley is a stay-at-home mom who homeschools her six children—all without a smartphone.

Folley sets up an environment for her kids—who range in age from two to eleven—where everyone learns together, with an emphasis on experiential learning and reading. She uses a Light Phone set up like a one-way pager. If someone sends her a text message, it is unlikely Folley will respond by text, opting to call or email the person instead. With the kids home a lot, especially in the colder months in Massachusetts, Folley intentionally keeps her Light Phone in another room.

"It's important to me to be very intentional about technology in my home because I really do not want them [the kids] to have the experience of being raised by screens or competing with a screen for my attention," she said.

Folley will often look around outside of the house and see distracted parents looking at screens with kids by their side.

"I witness that all the time, seeing how parents are drawn away from their children because of their devices and knowing how very fleeting childhood is and what an important role we play in our children's lives and how much our attention matters to them," she said.

Acquaintances will often push back, saying Folley's kids aren't learning how to use screens and will be at a disadvantage when they are older.

Folley isn't worried though. "The technologies are always becoming more intuitive. We don't even know what it's going to look like when they're coming of age. I just don't actually think that there's going to be any great learning curve."

The Folleys use the phone often in their house, but it's a landline. Deirdre enjoys watching her kids make calls to their grandmother, or seeing the younger ones pretend to make calls.

And she doesn't shy away from the topic of technology with her kids. When she's on the computer and they crowd around her to see what she's doing, she reminds them that the computer is a useful tool, but also one that sucks up a lot of time and doesn't bring happiness.

In addition to modeling what she sees as the right behavior for her kids, Folley and her husband ask guests not to use screens when they visit their home.

"I find that people are very respectful of that," she said. "Even people who I know pull it [their smartphone] out constantly do really make an effort when they're here to just keep it away. And my hope is that they will really appreciate their time here. I hope that our home is a place where good conversations happen and where people talk about things that matter, feel relaxed, and get a break."

My awareness of how much time I was spending on my phone soared when we had our first child. I remember taking Akiva to the zoo as a toddler; as he was watching the penguins waddle, I would be checking emails. As he got older, I saw how he would gravitate to the phone because I was on it all the time.

If we want to show our kids that we value time away from our screens, we need to emulate that behavior ourselves.

"Kids learn a lot more from what their parents do than what they say," said Dr. Clifford Sussman. "If you see your parent with their head in a cell phone while they're telling you to get off your video game, it's not a very strong, powerful message."

When I spoke to school principal Seth Lavin (see page 62) he told me that with more parents working remotely after the pandemic, kids experienced their parents being present and absent at the same time. He argues that in some ways, this can be worse than being absent because kids are accustomed to their parents being physically there, but not paying attention to them.

"If there's one very simplified piece of parenting advice I could give, it's never be on your phone when your kid is around," said Dr. Anna Lembke. "Because what happens is people disappear when they're on their phones and also they lose time. They have no conception of how long they've actually completely disappeared from their child."

Gaining Time

Joe Pankowski is a partner at Wofsey Rosen, a Connecticut law firm where he focuses on estate planning.

Pankowski remembers that when he was a fortysomething parent of two young kids, many of his friends and colleagues made the switch from basic phones to smartphones.

But Pankowski is different—he never owned a cell phone, period.

Part of his decision was work-driven. He'd seen firsthand that when other lawyers gave their cell phone number to clients it created an expectation that they were available even after work hours.

"That creates a really difficult feedback loop where a client will text you something, you text back, client has a follow-up, you text back, and all of a sudden your Saturday or Sunday is being soaked up by these texts which could have waited until Monday," he explained.

There was also a financial reality. If a client is billed at $525 an hour, that means an email or message that gets read automatically is charged at 0.1, or $52.50. If a message thread extends to a number of messages, the price can jump quickly.

"It will cost you [the client] an arm and a leg."

With the rise of email and texting, Pankowski was wary of how access to lawyers was unfolding. And then there was the personal side of it.

Pankowski would go out to dinner with his wife and see couples staring at their phones instead of each other. When he went to sports games with his kids, he would see parents staring down at their screens instead of enjoying the game. It was something he knew early on that he wanted to stay away from.

But then, in 2020, Pankowski gave in.

As a proud alumnus of Florida State University, Pankowski is a serious college football fan. Each fall, he travels from his home in Connecticut to Tallahassee for Seminoles games, and he catches them on the road in places like North Carolina, Massachusetts, and Pennsylvania.

Pankowski usually traveled with friends for these trips and, without a cell phone, would print out physical tickets for the games and for the air travel to get to them. Then in 2020, Florida State notified ticket holders that it was phasing out physical tickets and would require all fans to use digital tickets for games.

The move wasn't a shock to Pankowski—he was already struggling with buying tickets through outlets such as Ticketmaster and SeatGeek without a phone. So, in order to continue his rabid fandom of Seminoles football, Pankowski, then fifty-six, bought his first cell phone, an iPhone SE.

Because he'd seen how prevalent smartphone use had become among dear family and friends, he established guardrails from the start.

He decided to embrace the off-by-default philosophy.

When Pankowski first purchased his phone, he downloaded several apps, including StubHub, SeatGeek, and Ticketmaster in order to purchase Seminoles tickets. Eventually he would also download WhatsApp to connect over video chat every Sunday night with his two sons in California and Georgia. Otherwise, he committed to keeping his phone off.

His logic: "If you keep it turned off until you actually want to use it for something positive, it works, right?"

In addition to leaving his phone off, Pankowski never gives his cell phone number to clients. In fact, when I interviewed him for the first time in 2021, he told me that he didn't know his cell phone number by heart—and that was intentional.

"I don't want to give it out," he said. "I don't want them [clients] getting in touch with me off hours. There's a reason I have off hours."

Pankowski strives for face-to-face interactions in his practice. With his clients, he believes that nonverbal communication matters, and it saves them time and money compared to constant messaging.

When he sees a client cross their arms, he knows they might be disagreeing with him. Understanding facial expressions and body language is important in establishing any kind of relationship, he explained.

Having his smartphone off also gives Pankowski the time and space for productive meditation. He lives about a hundred yards from a dock, and kayaks year-round on the Long Island Sound. He takes his 45-pound orange kayak out almost every day at high tide, be it sunny, overcast, below freezing, or raining.

During the week, Pankowski likes to take the kayak out before work, when it's usually uncrowded and calm in the nearby estuary. He can see the seagulls flying overhead and will often stare at the fish swimming beside his kayak. If the tide is right, he also likes to go out at night to stare at the moon and stars.

It's the solitude Pankowski seeks, the time for self-reflection and what comes with it, including the space to solve problems. As he describes it, some of his best ideas as a lawyer surface from his time in the kayak.

But you don't need to have a kayak—going for a walk outside during lunch without a phone tethered to you can provide the same kind of effects that Pankowski gets. By limiting his phone to set activities—purchasing airfare and football tickets and having video calls with his kids—he has a system that allows him to turn his phone on only when he must.

And yet even without his smartphone on, Pankowski is easily reachable. Clients can call him on his work phone or send him an email. He uses Facebook as well as its messenger tool from his computer to stay in touch with friends from childhood and Florida State.

But those clients and friends also know that his cell phone isn't on. And that means when he's in a client meeting at work, or in the stands of a football game, or in his kayak, he is in the moment. He is present.

Not for the Faint of Heart

Sticking to the off-by-default philosophy for your detox may be more challenging than going to a basic phone. Keeping your smartphone off and only turning it on for critical tasks requires discipline and self-control. After your detox is finished, however, the off-by-default philosophy is one that I firmly believe you can stick with, though it can be loosened slightly.

Rather than only turning it on for critical tasks, we can change the definition of off-by-default to:

The default position of the smartphone should be off.
The only time the device should be turned on
*is to accomplish a task that **enhances your life**. After*
the task is complete, the phone is turned back off.

This reminds you that the smartphone is there to improve your life.

When I had my smartphone off for an entire year and had to decide what I was going to do after my detox was complete, the feeling of having my phone off was so profound that I didn't want to turn it back on.

I realized that there were certain aspects of my smartphone that I missed. I missed being able to use GPS for drives that were complicated. I liked being able to listen to a podcast while I did a monotonous chore, like dishes. I preferred getting a text with a code when I logged into a financial institution website, rather than having to call customer service.

Embracing the off-by-default philosophy, I realized that some weeks I can go days without ever turning on my smartphone.

I compare it to having a television. When you finish watching a show or a sporting event, you turn the TV off. You don't leave it on. So too with a smartphone: I find it is most useful in an off state.

The goal of the off-by-default philosophy is simple: By having your smartphone off, you will have control over the phone, rather than letting it have control over you.

GUIDELINES FOR OFF-BY-DEFAULT

When our phones are on, there is a part of our brain that is consciously or subconsciously thinking about them, according to experts. When we make the decision to leave our phones off, it changes the way our brain processes information. It gives us the space to allow our minds to focus on other experiences.

The off-by-default philosophy is one that resonates with Dr. Anna Lembke, who practices it herself. "When we power off the device, it's not just that we can't transmit, it's also that we can't receive," she said. "I think it changes our attention and changes our brainwaves such that we're no longer using a part of our brain, even unconsciously or subconsciously, to think about the phone and what it is receiving."

In the definition of the philosophy I presented earlier, I acknowledge there is some vagueness as to what "critical task" means. For your detox, I recommend being strict with the definition.

During your detox, here are examples of critical tasks where I would suggest turning on your phone:

- You printed out directions for a destination but are on the side of the highway lost. Rather than hitchhiking or walking miles to the nearest place to ask someone for directions, turn on your phone to use the GPS to get yourself back on track, then turn it off.

- You're out with your kids by yourself at the park and one of them gets hurt. You have to take them to urgent care but know that might mean getting home hours later than you expected. In the waiting room when you have a better sense of timing, ask the receptionist if you can use the office phone to make a call. If they say no, turn on your phone to let your partner know what happened, then turn it off again. You don't want to make someone worried sick about you if you were supposed to be home in the afternoon and aren't home until after bedtime.

- A transformer blew near your house and you've lost power. It's nighttime and the temperatures are below freezing outside. You want to alert your local utility company. Turn on your phone to alert them, then turn it back off.
- There is a serious car accident in front of you and both drivers are injured. After checking on them, go to your car and turn on your phone to dial 911.

Here are a few scenarios where you definitely shouldn't turn on your phone:

- You're at a concert with your friends and want to grab a video or photos of the band. Don't turn your phone on. Be in the moment.
- Your child is having a meltdown in public, and you want to use your phone to show a movie to calm them down. Don't turn it on.
- You're out to lunch with work colleagues and disagree about when the movie *That Thing You Do!* was released. Don't turn on your smartphone to look it up. (And it was 1996, if you're curious!)
- You're at the airport in the terminal and there are significant delays. Don't turn on your phone.

In the end you'll be left with your best judgment during your detox, but afterward, once you've experienced just how enhanced your focus has become, it will get easier to make the right call. Keep in mind that this process, at first, is supposed to be uncomfortable. But once you get past this initial stage, the reward will be well worth it.

Option 3: Getting Rid of Your Phone

There are forty-eight mountains in New Hampshire that exceed 4,000 feet in elevation.

Along the often-formidable trails to reach these summits, it's common to find hikers using trekking poles to assist with uneven, rocky terrain and head-lamps to pierce the predawn darkness. For Stephen Kurczy, he carried one more piece of extra "baggage": his one-year-old son, Mansfield.

With his son strapped to his back, Kurczy managed to join an elite group of hikers—the 4,000-footers club, or those who climbed all forty-eight mountains. But what makes his story relevant here is something that he chooses not to carry with him on hikes.

His cell phone. Because he doesn't own one.

After graduating from college in 2005, Kurczy started working as a journalist, first in Connecticut and then in New York City. Before leaving in 2007 for a job in Cambodia, Kurczy remembers sitting in Brooklyn's Prospect Park with a group of friends. They huddled together as one of them took out a first-generation iPhone. She started to google various things as the group aahed over how much information was available in such a portable way. The experience left an impression on Kurczy.

In the summer of 2009, after two years in Cambodia, Kurczy was planning to travel across Asia for a few months before settling back in the United States. His five-year-old Samsung flip phone wasn't working well. When he realized that it wouldn't be functional for his travels, Kurczy decided to throw it away.

Although he was frustrated with his basic phone—how it was by his side when he went to bed and then greeted him in the morning with new messages from his editor—the impetus for getting rid of it had little to do with how much space it occupied in his life. Rather, he would be traveling, and since the clunky phone was on its last legs, he figured he'd just get a new one when he returned home to the States.

He figured wrong.

When Kurczy arrived in Boston in early 2010 for a job at the *Christian Science Monitor*, he still didn't have a cell phone. Now that he was back in a major city, Kurczy remembers deliberating over when to walk into the Apple Store to buy his first smartphone.

Yet something held him back. He knew that once he walked in, salespeople would approach him and explain how much better his life would be with a smartphone, drawing him into the Apple product culture that was becoming more and more ubiquitous.

Kurczy walked into the store twice to explore the offerings—and each time came out "frustrated." Days became weeks and weeks became months and Kurczy still didn't have a cell phone, even a basic one.

"It began as a personal choice to avoid getting a cell phone for a while. But I faced so much pressure to get a device from my bosses, friends, and family, that I had to actively refuse to get one," he told me.

Writing for a major news publication in an era when many journalists were establishing themselves on social media and more content was being pushed online, not having a cell phone was in "constant tension" with Kurczy's work.

"I really bucked that societal pressure to get a device," he said. "I didn't like people telling me what to do, especially with a device that seemed to be not for my sake, but for *their* sake. Like people saying, 'You need to be in touch, so I can be in touch with you.' And me saying, 'Hang on, I thought I had some autonomy over my life.'"

At the recommendation of his colleagues, Kurczy did ultimately sign up for a Twitter account. But because he didn't have a smartphone, he felt his social media usage was under control. When he left the newsroom, his Twitter activity stayed at the office.

"The smartphone is the device that enables social media to have a constant influence and hold over your life. So the two are much connected in my mind," he said.

When Kurczy moved to Brazil in 2013 as a foreign correspondent, he remained resolute, and still did not get a phone.

How did he pull it off? He primarily used Google Voice to make calls from his laptop.

"It's not that I'm a technophobe," Kurczy told me. "It's that I don't want to have 24-7 access to this device. I don't want it to have 24-7 access to me in part because I know that I would abuse it. This stuff is meant to be addictive. It's built to be addictive."

By the time Kurezy moved back to New York in 2016, smartphone consumption nationwide was at an even higher level.

Love, Offline

On a train ride back home to Connecticut over Labor Day weekend, Kurczy ran into Jenna Cho, whom he had worked with at a newspaper ten years earlier. They were on a train platform in New Haven, both looking for the Shore Line East, a local track, to get home for the weekend. They got on the same train and enjoyed talking with each other. When Cho arrived at her destination, Kurczy wanted to stay in touch and, with little time to explain, told Cho that he would send her a message.

"It was too complicated to try and go through the whole process of saying, 'I don't have a cell phone, here's why,'" he explained.

"He never asked me for my number," Cho recalled. "So I thought that was a little bit odd, and when he did message me, it was on Twitter via direct message.

And I think that's when I learned that he didn't have a cell phone."

So, how would Kurczy and Cho cultivate a relationship when one partner didn't have a cell phone in 2016? To start out, Kurczy and Cho messaged each other over Twitter. Eventually, they transitioned to iMessage, which Kurczy could use from his laptop with his Apple account. When they went out on dates, they had to be intentional about where exactly they would meet and at what time since Kurczy couldn't be reached once he left his home.

Cho told me that past relationships she had been in were very text heavy, but since Kurczy didn't have patience for all of the messaging from a computer, much of their interaction was face-to-face.

"It sounds kind of bizarre," he said, laughing. "But obviously it was just like how we all used to meet up fifteen years ago."

And it worked out: They eventually got married.

. . . . .

The intentionality that both Kurczy and Cho showed while dating has carried over as they parent their two children. When Kurczy goes on long hikes with his kids, he goes through contingency plans with Cho for picking them up with the car.

"It forces us in that moment to be extra thoughtful about planning ahead. It also amps up the responsibility on me to make it successful. I can't be slacking off here because my wife's waiting."

For some of the more strenuous hikes, like a fifty-five-mile one he did, he'll tell Cho: "If you don't see me by this time, that means there's a problem. If you don't see me by this time, that means you should call for rescue."

I asked Cho what this dynamic is like for her, and what her mindset is when he takes their kids on all-day hikes without a cell phone.

"It isn't the fact that he doesn't have a phone that is worrisome," Cho said. "There are times when I wish that he packed a little bit more, but I also understand the fact that he has a kid backpack, which is already heavy as it is, plus the kid, plus diapers, wipes, and foods. There's only so much you can carry. So yeah, it isn't really the cell phone that I'm worried about."

Have there been moments for Kurczy where his not having a cell phone have made things more difficult for Cho?

Absolutely. He recalls his fortieth birthday, when he and Cho went away together on a ski trip in northern Vermont. He was out skiing early in the morning while Cho was still in their room at the resort looking for her ski pass so she could meet up with some friends. She searched frantically for the pass and knew that Kurczy would likely know where it was. But without a way to contact him, she had to tell her friends to go skiing without her.

"That was a frustrating moment, obviously. That could have been resolved by just me having a cell phone and checking it throughout the day. At the same time, she knew she couldn't message me and that it wasn't going to work out," he said.

"I remember being really annoyed," Cho told me in a separate conversation about that experience. "Because we got a big dump of snow the night before. . . . It was just a stupid logistical thing that was keeping me from going out. But it worked out," she said, explaining that when Kurczy got back to the room, he found her ski pass.

Although that memory stuck out to Kurczy, for Cho, she doesn't find those moments to be all that problematic. If she had to pinpoint the most challenging aspect about Kurczy not having a cell phone, it is everyone assuming that she can be "the personal messenger for everything that needs to be communicated to Steve."

For a birthday party in Kurczy's family, she gets the message. For visits to the pediatrician, she receives the alerts. For preschool and daycare, Cho is the emergency contact and is the one getting text messages with pictures and updates throughout the day.

Kurczy admits that his not having a phone puts more responsibility on Cho, but he remains steadfast in his beliefs. "We should all have the choice to be able to live without a cell phone and to not necessarily be set back from our interactions with society in significant ways."

He is also realistic about his decision and the impact it has. "I've taken myself out of a lot of the modern-day economy," he confides. "And it makes me all the more convinced to not have a cell phone and to continue sticking out my elbows to try and create some space for other people who don't want to have these devices."

That Kurczy doesn't have a cell phone hasn't stopped him from getting involved in his community. He is a member of his local volunteer fire department. When he signed up and was going through the onboarding process, he was told that he would need to use a smartphone and download an app to get real-time responses for fire alerts. The app allows the fire station to know where he is, and how long it will take to get to the fire station.

When Kurczy explained that he didn't have a cell phone, the fire department issued him a pager, which he carries with him when he leaves the house so that he can be notified when there is an alert.

"I think I am the only person in the entire fire department who does not have a smartphone," he admitted.

Cho told me that Kurczy's habits have definitely rubbed off on her. After meeting him, she decided to always leave her phone on silent when she goes out of the house, wanting to be more present and less distracted by her phone.

She also deleted her social media accounts on Facebook, Twitter, and Instagram.

"I've given all those up, and not because he asked me to, not because he suggested or anything, but because it made me question why I was not questioning," she said.

In addition to hiking, one of Kurczy's favorite activities is rock climbing. He finds the experience to be restorative, pushing out any negative thoughts or emotions. When he returns home after a climb, he feels like a different person.

"Imagine if I had a smartphone in my pocket and it started ringing when I'm halfway up the wall—what a break from this wonderfully intense moment in my life."

When kids came into the picture, Kurczy became even more convinced that he had made the right decision to not have a phone.

"If I don't want my kid to be holding a smartphone all the time, then I'd better not have a smartphone," he said.

Cho owns two smartphones—one for work and another for personal use—and Kurczy believes his decision balances things between the two of them. "It provides a little bit of, like, example for our kids as they're growing up about how we would like them to approach technology with a bit more distance to not make it so central in their lives," he said.

Cho describes their home as being pretty typical: They still have Wi-Fi and their laptops, and at times, she said they aren't the best role models in terms of putting their devices away, even with Kurczy not having a cell phone.

The kids often watch cartoons in the morning, and enjoy looking at photos on Kurczy's iPod or Cho's smartphone.

But, as both explained to me, they are present with their kids.

Most people would be shocked to hear that a millennial doesn't carry a cell phone. But if you look at Kurczy, with a career as a professor at Providence College in Rhode Island, a wife, two kids, a passion for high-quality leisure activities, and an investment in community, you'd think to yourself, *Why can't I do something like this?*

"That initially trivial decision to throw away my device [in Cambodia] has turned into this kind of conviction that my life is no worse for not having a cell phone, and is arguably better," he told me.

"He takes me on many interesting adventures and it's never boring," Cho said. "I admire that a lot. . . . I'm willing to trade sometimes the annoyance of not being able to text him. I'd rather have that than be with a partner who is constantly on his phone."

Recognize You Are the Exception and Be Transparent

One of the most important things to realize when you are doing your detox is how your decision might impact others. Understand that when you break up with your phone and establish a more balanced relationship with it, the rest of the world is likely on a different wavelength. If you make plans with someone and there isn't a way to get in touch if you have a flat tire or are running late, that could turn someone off to either working with you or simply being your friend.

But if you establish in advance that there won't be a way to get in touch with you, or that you don't have WhatsApp, you can avoid burning bridges.

When writer Kate Emmons, whom we met in the off-by-default section earlier, went through her detox, she messaged people privately as well as on social media with the following:

"I'm embracing life without a smartphone, so instead of a text I would love it if you reached out to me via email or phone call, because I would love to take the time to connect with you in a more personal way. I would love to know how you're doing . . . and not just a 'status update.'"

In the story that follows about Steve Hilton, a former senior adviser to United Kingdom prime minister David Cameron from 2010 to 2012, the requirement to be upfront with people before you start your detox is particularly resonant.

Several years after moving to the United States following his government work in the UK, Hilton launched his own talk show on Fox News. He has interviewed a former president in the Rose Garden, grilled political pundits, and posed tough questions to cabinet members. Now the founder of a nonpartisan think tank and a podcast host, most people don't realize that Hilton doesn't use a smartphone. In fact, for many years, he didn't own a phone at all.

When Hilton relocated to the United States in 2012, his government-issued flip phone no longer worked. Without a cell phone, he had to decide whether he would get a new one. He opted not to.

Life without a phone brought with it many benefits, but one of the biggest challenges was not being able to easily connect to his family while traveling. For years, Hilton would use hotel room phones as a way to call his wife and two young kids. But over time, room phones became less dependable, and many hotels charged heavily for long-distance calls.

Hilton considered this an inconvenience and ended up buying a flip phone because he couldn't justify the expense of the hotel charges. But he would only turn it on a dozen or so times a year when he was traveling. He told me that he doesn't refer to it as a phone, rather as a "family connection device."

Because Hilton is so plugged in to the political world but so infrequently picks up his basic phone, the responsibility to proactively communicate with individuals he plans to meet falls squarely on his shoulders.

"If it's someone I don't know and I am meeting them for the first time for a business meeting . . . I'm very conscious of putting myself in their shoes and their assumption that I have a phone," he told me.

"Therefore, if they're late or want to change the venue, they'll assume that they can get in touch with you. So, it's on *me* to tell them that that's not possible and to alert them."

He added that it is important to accept the fact that if

someone can't get in touch with you or is massively delayed and needs to make a change, you won't be informed. He told me that it's hardly ever happened, even in all of his years of networking.

When Hilton lets people know that he doesn't use a cell phone, he's typically asked, "How do you operate? How do you ever meet up with anyone? How do you do this?"

Hilton explains the benefits of his approach to others, but emphasizes that "it's on me to make it work because *I'm the exception*, I'm choosing to do that."

Hilton would eventually get a smartphone. His wife, a top executive at Netflix, told him that she felt the pressure was always on her to take pictures when they went out as a family, which meant she had to be on her phone even more.

Hilton bought a standalone camera but had trouble connecting it to the cloud. When he got his own smartphone he removed the SIM card, and now refers to it as "the camera."

"It isn't used for any other purpose," he said.

Going All In

The decision to not carry a cell phone at all for your entire detox will likely be the most difficult adjustment of all the breakup styles. However, it could very well be the most impactful in how you reestablish your relationship with your smartphone.

It might just come down to your level of conviction when you start. If you feel very strongly and want to go all in on the detox, or if you want to get a sense of what life is truly like without a phone, don't carry one at all.

Although Stephen Kurczy has been without a phone for more than a decade, you only really have to do it for two months during your own detox.

According to a 2024 report from the Pew Research Center, the number of cell phone users continues to rise, with 99 percent of people between the ages of 18 and 49 owning a cell phone. For those between the ages of 50 and 64, 98 percent own one.

The stats are clear—the number of people who don't own cell phones is dwindling. For those who feel strongly about not having a phone, like Kurczy, it can become a part of your identity.

As it is for Stefan Syski, a database manager and history teacher at a private school outside of Washington, DC, who has been without a cell phone since 2009.

Syski purchased a basic phone for his last year of law school at The George Washington University, but after he graduated, he found that he wasn't using the phone very much, so eventually he got rid of it.

Syski, who did computer programming as an adolescent, understood at an early age that he liked to be in control over the technology around him. A husband and father of ten children, Syski has to be very intentional with the time he has. When he is not working at school, Syski's number one priority is his family, so when he's home he wants his focus to be on them.

"The one thing that I've tried to do with my wife over our married life is to shape our desire for what is good in life," he shared with me. "If you're thinking about wanting to shape your goals and choose what is right . . . then you're going to put the things away from you that will distract and take you in the wrong direction."

When Syski tells people, including his students, that he doesn't have a cell phone most don't believe him. But Syski is still plenty reachable. He has an email address, work phone number, home phone number, and a Google Voice number so he can receive text messages to log into various platforms. For their home landline, Syski purchased a Gabb phone, a portable phone with no internet, that makes calls and sends texts. With his oldest child at fourteen, Syski wanted his kids to be comfortable sending texts so that when they eventually leave home, they would have that skill.

For Syski, one of the more useful aspects of not having a cell phone has been training himself to be very strong at understanding directions, so he doesn't have to be dependent on GPS. In addition, he enjoys carrying around a Moleskine notebook where he enters calendar entries, notes, and appointments.

"That's sort of the way I feel order," he told me.

GUIDELINES FOR GETTING RID OF YOUR PHONE

When you are ready to decommission your phone, here are a few options:

- Go to your local mobile carrier store or a place like Best Buy and recycle it. You might even get some money back.

- Make it a party. Gather a group of family and friends for a night of farewells to your smartphone. Write a speech. Two side benefits to throwing a party with others: It will increase accountability to stick to your detox and may encourage a friend or two to reconsider their own relationship with their smartphone.

- As popularized by the 1999 Mike Judge film *Office Space*, find a safe, open area, put on protective eyewear, and use your favorite bat to show your smartphone how it has made you feel.

- By getting rid of your phone and mobile plan, you will be saving money. Therefore, take family or friends out to a nice meal. At the end of the evening, choose one of the options above.

Option 4: Quitting with Someone Else

Technology always played a big part in Ella Jones's life.

Growing up in the United Kingdom with a father who was a technology professional, Jones was exposed to screens at an early age. By the time she turned twelve, she'd saved up enough money to buy her first smartphone, a Samsung Galaxy. She quickly gravitated to using social media, and when she purchased a used iPhone at fourteen, it vastly expanded her options—she could now download all the popular social media apps that her friends used.

As a teen, her level of screen consumption increased when her school gave each student an iPad.

"I think they were trying to be really tech forward at the time. And that basically led to the whole school being very screwed into screens in terms of games, social media, everything," she told me. And with that came the social pressure and expectation that everyone would be on their devices.

When Jones started college at the University of Leeds in 2019, she started meeting new friends and noticed that people weren't asking for her phone number to get in touch, but rather for her Snapchat or Instagram handle.

Group chats quickly started among peers, as well as Facebook groups for all of the various clubs. She had to download Facebook Messenger to keep up with her social life.

When the coronavirus pandemic came, everything at school went remote, and Jones moved back to her parents' house, at which point, "My phone usage just went straight through the roof," she told me. She would spend two straight hours scrolling, then as if snapping out of a trance she'd wonder, "What am I doing?"

At the same time she was also maintaining a long-distance relationship with her boyfriend, Joe Wakley. The two met in high school when they sat next to each other in geography class. "I thought the girl next to her was very attractive, so I tried to chat her up and it didn't work," Wakley recalled, laughing. But Jones had taken notice of him and sent him a couple of messages, and the two began to date.

Wakley left the United Kingdom for college, attending Queens University in Belfast, Northern Ireland, a one-hour flight from Jones in Leeds.

Ever since he got his first smartphone when he was a teenager, Wakley described his relationship with it as "uncomfortable." But it wasn't until college that he began to really reflect on his relationship with it. He realized that the expectation from others to respond to messages quickly was causing issues in his life.

"Any time my phone would ring during the day, I'd have a bit of a like, 'Ugh,' annoyance reaction. I'd just, like, chuck it in the back of my bag and turn it off. And all these new friends who I'm making, they're all like, 'Oh, you never respond to your texts, please respond.'"

During his second year of college, Wakley's uncle, who lived nearby, told him about a group of monks who worked with students on campus to help build community.

The brothers were a part of the New Monasticism movement, a group of Christians who emphasize prayer, communal life, and contemplation.

The brothers invited Wakley and his roommates to live with them for three weeks. Wanting to open themselves up to new experiences, Wakley and his friends decided to leave the comfort of their house to learn something and be exposed to a way of life different from theirs.

Living with the brothers from the monastery was an eye-opening experience for Wakley. He and his friends still attended classes as they had before, but each morning and evening was filled with contemplation. There was morning prayer each day, and the evening was for dialogue and reflection. Wakley and his friends slept on the floor and ate simple foods.

They noticed that all the brothers carried basic phones, leading to a house environment that was not screen dependent. Wakley left the experience impressed and remembered saying to himself: "I want a life that's simpler, that's slower, that's more peaceful."

When he moved back to his house for the rest of the semester, his roommates were using their smartphones the way they had before. But for Wakley, there was something about embracing a more intentional life that resonated deeply.

After thinking about it for a month, he switched the SIM card over from his smartphone to a Nokia basic phone. He didn't tell Jones about the change, deciding instead to wait and tell her when he visited her in Leeds for her birthday a few weeks later.

But Wakley's plan wasn't just to tell her, it was to convince her to do the same.

Breaking Up, Together

Ilkley Moor is a popular West Yorkshire destination for its walking trails and panoramic views near Leeds. Wakley and Jones went there for a hike, walking across a wide grassland. It was a sunny autumn day, clear enough to look out across the expansive, tall plateaus that surrounded them.

Taking in the moment, Wakley thought about the best way to broach the smartphone topic with Jones. It wasn't just that he wanted to tell her that he turned off his smartphone—he very much hoped they could find a way to do it together, that she would want that too.

Wakley yearned for that feeling of community and togetherness the brothers had in Belfast; he wanted that kind of closeness with the love of his life. On the hike, Jones pulled out her smartphone and sent a text message. Slightly irked, Wakley felt if there was any moment to bring it up, now was the time.

"Ella is very determined . . . she won't do something if you just tell her to do something, which is something I love in her," Wakley said. "But she does respond very well to questions. . . . So I just raised the question: 'Why do you think you need that smartphone?'"

Jones started going through her phone app by app and, after talking it through with Wakley, concluded that most of the things she wanted to do on her phone could be accomplished just as easily on her laptop.

"I realized, 'Oh, I can access social media on my laptop, so I don't need it in my pocket at all times,'" she said. "I can just check it on Safari or whatever I'm using instead of having that kind of constant buzz in my pocket."

After going through every app of the smartphone one by one, Jones realized that the only parts of the smartphone she felt like she really needed were WhatsApp and Facebook because clubs on campus used both for messaging.

Wakley told her that she could get a simpler phone that supports apps, and only download those two, making her use of the phone more intentional and less addictive than her current smartphone.

What made the prospect of not having a smartphone more appealing for Jones was that Wakley would be doing it too.

"There was an interesting dynamic there, because I knew he was doing it as well. So it was less of the FOMO and more of a challenge that we both did."

That evening, Jones ordered a Nokia 2720 Flip phone.

Wakley flew back to Belfast, thrilled that he'd accomplished what he wanted—Jones would be going through this experience with him. They would do it together.

.....

Simplifying their phones changed the dynamic of Wakley and Jones's long-distance relationship, for the better.

Rather than FaceTiming and texting throughout the day like they did before, Wakley and Jones called each other once or twice a week. They would sometimes go a day or two at a time without talking, but the conversations they had were longer and carried greater meaning, what Wakley described as having "a healthier balance."

Although they would sometimes send each other silly videos or messages over text, the practice of messaging fizzled out, in part due to how cumbersome it was to text on their basic phones. They wanted to spend their time communicating "deliberately and intentionally."

With the phone less enticing, Jones rekindled her love of reading. She also liked that before going somewhere new she would have to write down the directions, jotting them down on a sticky note that she attached to her dashboard.

"It's so funny because you think that that's just a really annoying thing," she told me. "But actually it really helped with my navigational skills . . . I have so much better awareness of where I live and how to get places than whenever I use GPS all the time."

After graduating from college, Jones moved to Belfast to be with Wakley. Following a nine-month detox from her smartphone, she made the decision to turn it back on. In moving to a new city there were a number of things for which she felt she needed a smartphone, including public transportation.

Because of the detox, however, she was able to find a healthier balance.

Professionally, Jones is a digital content manager, and social media strategy is a primary part of her work. She decided to keep her business and personal digital footprints separate by keeping a work phone and a personal phone.

When she goes to work, she uses her work phone and has access to all of the bells and whistles you'd expect from a smartphone, including social media applications. When she is done with work she puts her work phone away and uses her personal smartphone, which doesn't have social media.

For Wakley, his detox lasted a year and a half before he got an iPhone as a work device at his education policy job. The process of bringing a smartphone back into his life was challenging. He described the experience as "readdiction very quickly." The barriers Wakley had built around his smartphone broke down: He started streaming video on his phone regularly, spending too much of his time with YouTube Shorts.

Wakley started to hate his smartphone again. He decided to use it for work only—after work was over, he'd swap the SIM card over to his basic phone.

For Wakley and Jones, turning off their smartphones and then turning them back on has brought them closer. It has brought accountability.

Reflecting on the whole detox experience, Jones said she feels that technology can be a barrier to social interaction and the ability to love others.

One month after my interviews with them in 2023, they got married. That's love.

Get Comfortable without GPS

Jen Wasserstein is an immigration attorney with a law practice based in Washington, DC. Originally from the United States, Wasserstein has lived abroad since 2010, first in Morocco, then in Italy, and now Spain. When she lived in the United States she used a basic phone, but when she first moved abroad she got rid of her phone and was without one for three years.

In 2013, Wasserstein would eventually purchase another basic phone, but those three phoneless years were instrumental in how she rewrote her relationship with the technology.

"I really loved being without a phone," she told me.

The motivation for getting a new phone was her daughter getting older: Wasserstein wanted to be more available if something came up.

She purposely didn't choose a smartphone because she wanted to keep that feeling of being "untethered" when she left the house. With emails from clients pouring in all day, as well as connections through Skype, she treasured that feeling of not being able to check messages when she was away from home. "If there's an emergency at the office, I don't know about it. It's kind of nice," she said.

Having lived in three different foreign countries over the last decade, I was most interested to learn how Wasserstein coped without a GPS.

She told me that she'll often look up new places on her computer before she goes somewhere and then write down the directions. If her destination is near somewhere that she's familiar with, she'll jot it down.

She also carries a paper map of her town, Valencia, Spain, in her purse. Ditto for Rome when she lived there. She also isn't afraid to ask people for help if she gets lost, whether it's someone from the post office or a delivery person.

"I have a terrible sense of direction and I get lost constantly," she told me, laughing. "But I really don't mind because I'll meet someone nice who will tell me which way to go."

Saul Pwanson, a software engineer from Seattle (see page 153), described going to Amsterdam and then Budapest for work without a functioning smartphone. In addition to not being able to connect as easily with work colleagues, he also had to navigate two unfamiliar cities. And though it admittedly took him a little longer to get places, he eventually found his way.

"I figured it out," he told me. "I learned my surroundings better than if I'd had a smartphone."

Like Wasserstein, Pwanson would often ask people for directions, and even with a language barrier he managed to get what he needed.

"It was actually kind of nice to engage with somebody," he said.

Pwanson described the experience as "empowering," saying that he felt really good about himself because he was able to find his way around foreign cities on his own. When he's home in Seattle, he tends to write out directions on a note card, which forces him "to engage with the directions before I've left." He admitted that he has always been terrible with directions, but feels that he is better at them now because he writes them down more often.

Quitting as a Way to Connect More Deeply

Anthony Donataccio was a successful business-man in Australia, working his way up from retail management to a senior role at a boutique wealth management firm as a finance manager. Donataccio described his phone usage in his career as "intense," with emails and phone calls coming across his personal and work phones around the clock.

"He was very wired in, and it was quite toxic," said his wife, Michele Perry, a book editor. "It was just 24-7 for him. His phone was on all the time."

Eventually Donataccio and Perry, who were both still in their thirties, decided that life was moving too fast. So in 2015 they began traveling the world together, renting homes in other countries for several months at a time, with Italy as their home base.

As they found themselves in unfamiliar places, they couldn't miss a similarity to what they saw in Australia: how hooked people were to their phones. Sitting in restaurants in Malaysia or Thailand, Donataccio remembers looking at other couples glued to their phones, not uttering a word to each other for an entire meal.

During their travels, they'd regularly meet interesting people who introduced them to new perspectives. One topic that came up repeatedly in their conversations was the issue of surveillance.

As world travelers, Donataccio and Perry were using their smartphones a lot. Soon, they began to wonder about their own privacy and security.

Then 2020 came, and Italy was one of the first countries to lock down during the pandemic. Envisioning how much more government surveillance would occur as a result, Donataccio and Perry decided that they would purchase basic phones for themselves online. When the phones arrived in the mail, they immediately switched the SIM cards from their smartphones over.

Donataccio described the first week of their not having smartphones as tricky, since so many of their personal and professional habits revolved around the device. Donataccio recalls the first few times leaving his home with his basic phone and being in a panic that he forgot to bring it because of how much lighter it felt in his pocket.

The first time he and Perry went out to lunch without their smartphones, they learned they had to order food by scanning a QR code to see the menu. They explained to the restaurant staff that they didn't have smartphones and a list of the menu items that was pinned to a board in the kitchen was brought to their table.

Perry thought to herself: "This is crazy. How can you not have menus anymore?"

But soon enough, things started falling into place for them.

Soon after they switched to basic phones, Donataccio and Perry embarked on an experiment in order to better acquaint themselves with their new reality. They took a day trip from their home in Tuscany to Liguria, an Italian region to which they had never been before.

Without smartphones and the use of GPS technology, the hour-plus train ride was eye-opening.

"Anthony and I sit down, and we look at each other and go, 'Oh, this is nice, isn't it?' Looking at what people are doing, having a bit of a chat together, looking out the window of the train, watching the world go by. It's all very lovely. No one else was doing that," she told me.

Donataccio and Perry used paper maps instead of Google Maps. If they had a question, they asked people on the street instead of looking at their phones. Even the experience of eating changed, because they weren't distracted.

It made Donataccio realize "how much experience of visiting that place we would've lost had we relied so much on the phone."

When they came back that night, they realized that they had spoken to each other and remembered more about their trip than any other they'd taken together over the last five years.

Donataccio and Perry began to realize that although they initially unplugged for privacy reasons, what they were really getting was a more focused life together.

"Like with any experiment," Donataccio explained, "you might be looking for an objective or a result, but then you discover so much other stuff as a result of that as well."

Donataccio and Perry at one point bought walkie-talkies so they could easily contact each other without using a phone when they walked or rode bikes in the neighborhood. Perry's parents, who moved to nearby Lucca, also got walkie-talkies, as did friends from Arizona who moved to Italy. Donataccio described it as a "cool way to communicate."

He believes what made their phone reset such a success was that he was able to do it with his lifelong partner by his side, supporting each other along the way. And his relationship with Perry grew as a part of the process. "Because we don't have our phone in our hands doing the stuff that we used to do . . . we're definitely spending more present time together," he said.

Whether it's eating dinner together at home or watching a television show, Donataccio told me he feels a strong connection, describing his relationship with Perry as unique. "We have this ability to not even communicate verbally and understand each other," he said.

GUIDELINES FOR QUITTING WITH SOMEONE ELSE

Duos like Wakley and Jones or Donataccio and Perry show what a detox can look like when someone else is along for the ride. It isn't a requirement, of course, but it does have the advantage of making the process that much more of a team effort and therefore more likely to succeed. I was lucky to have a strong support system around me, but I can only imagine how much more energized by the process I would have been if I'd done it with someone else.

"I think that when you have another person there, I think there is something psychologically more motivating to that," said Dr. Michael Fraser, a screen addiction specialist who serves as the director of the Child Adolescent Outpatient Clinic at Lincoln Medical Center in the Bronx.

As you're planning your own smartphone detox, consider approaching someone in your circle to do it with. Be it a spouse, friend, or family member, going through a detox with someone else just makes it that much more enticing.

"The most important thing from birth on, is attachment," said Dr. Hilarie Cash. "That is the thing that is foundational for us all."

Cash explains that when you're with someone you care about who also takes care of you, it releases neurochemicals in our brains that keep us regulated. Whereas the internet produces an adverse effect, what Cash describes as the "illusion of attachment."

"If we can go on a detox and get into the zone of a new lifestyle, and we can do it with somebody . . . that's the ideal," she said.

"It's so counter-cultural," Dr. Anna Lembke told me. "But if you have somebody else who's doing it with you, it's like a touch-stone where you can validate it and say, 'No, this is a good thing that I'm doing it together with this other person.' And of course we need that because there's so much messaging that tells us that we're really weird if we don't have a smartphone."

Doing a detox with just a spouse or friend isn't the only option—it can also be done as a family unit. Dr. Clifford Sussman is a big believer in families detoxing together. When he's working with a young adult dealing with a screen addiction, he tries to create a system where his client doesn't feel like they're being singled out, but rather supported during the detox.

"We're social creatures," Sussman told me. "We're more likely to do what the people around us are doing. And then you don't feel as isolated."

In order to make your detox with someone else a success, here are some tips to follow:

- **Goals:** Whether it's in a shared Google Doc or on a piece of physical paper, write down your goals and what you're both hoping to get out of the process. Stick it on your fridge to serve as a constant reminder of why you are doing this together.

- **Check-ins:** Schedule a set time at least once a week to talk about what you are going through and feeling. If you feel yourself struggling the first week or two, be sure to communicate that. The other person might be feeling the same way.

- **Scheduled Activities:** Make plans several times a week for screen-free activities. This could involve going for a walk, visiting a museum, or eating at a restaurant. Without a phone in the picture, these experiences will be highly rewarding, and you will be doing them together.

CHAPTER 4

Newfound Time

You've successfully embraced a breakup style and now find yourself with hours of additional time each day. The next question naturally is: How are you going to spend it?

Your mind will crave high-dopamine replacement activities. At home, you might be tempted to scroll social media, online shop, or stream television most of the night. At work, you might gravitate to internet surfing or incessant email inbox refreshes.

Resist those temptations.

Giving yourself space and solitude can be unsettling, but in this chapter you'll learn how to meaningfully fill your time. I will present four key life areas to focus on for your detox: work, relationships, screen-free hobbies, and the self.

All of this is a way of reinventing yourself. It's what makes the detox process rewarding.

Let's get started.

Work

....

The studio lights glare down on a board with sixty-four squares and thirty-two pieces.

It might be frigid outside on this December day, but inside the 1 Hotel in downtown Toronto, things are heating up. A yearlong season and points race have come down to this moment, to two of the world's greatest competitors vying for a $200,000 prize. From India to the United States, hundreds of thousands of people are streaming the event. It's the 2023 Champions Chess Tour Finals.

Thanks to the popularity of the 2020 Netflix mini-series *The Queen's Gambit*, as well as a pandemic that forced most people indoors for long stretches, chess popularity grew worldwide, with millions joining Chess.com in 2020 alone.

In Toronto this afternoon, Norway's Magnus Carlsen sits on one side of the board. A five-time world champion by the age of thirty-three, Carlsen had cemented his legacy next to Garry Kasparov as one of the greatest chess players of all time. Across from him is thirty-year-old American grand master Wesley So, one of the top ten chess players in the world and a worthy opponent to Carlsen.

The broadcasters covering the event acknowledge that the underdog is So, who sits poised, adjusting his pieces carefully on the board before the match starts.

He then takes off his glasses and removes a ring from his left hand, putting them to the side of the board. He focuses as Carlsen hits the chess clock, starting the match.

On the surface, So is like many of his chess peers. He's popular among fans and a fighter, playing aggressive moves and establishing solid positions. But what separates So from everyone else is a decision he made eight years prior.

. . . . .

So grew up in the Philippines and learned chess from his father. He would go to the park as a kid, bring a chess board, and challenge anyone willing to play.

He loved the game and started playing competitively in tournaments at a young age, eventually becoming the then-youngest player to pass the 2600 rating (a measure of a player's probable performance) in 2008, a record previously held by Carlsen. So reached number 80 in the world rankings as a teen and was considered a phenom and a rare talent.

But as So competed in chess tournaments from Europe to Asia, most people didn't realize that he wasn't just battling his opponents over the board—he was also fighting internal demons. When So completed school as a sixteen-year-old he was living in Manila by himself, with his biological parents settled in Canada. He got into bad relationships with friends and was addicted to computer games. He also started drinking alcohol. And his game suffered.

"That's part of the reason why my chess wasn't improving," he told me.

So's world ranking started to slip. As much as he wanted to believe in himself and his ability, he couldn't, not quite.

"I thought I was going to be okay," he said. "I thought I could make it. But looking back, it's clear I wasn't going to be successful. No chance at all . . . I didn't have the discipline and the support."

So self-describes as having a "very addictive personality," one that too often found comfort in unproductive screen time. He often used his phone before going to bed and would stay up far longer than he wanted.

Still, as a top 100 player, So received scholarship offers from American universities who were recruiting him to play on their chess teams. He knew he would have to leave the Philippines if he wanted to reach his potential as one of the world's best chess players.

Without much money and not knowing what to expect in a new country, So decided to take a leap of faith and in 2012 accepted an offer to attend Webster University outside of St. Louis, Missouri.

So described the experience of starting college at Webster as challenging, but the change of scenery was a refreshing chance to start anew and "let go of the past." The Webster chess team was also loaded with strong talent from all over the world. But as much as So enjoyed the competition, he still hadn't realized his true potential.

Then in 2014, something clicked, and So went from being a grand master to one of the top ten players in the world.

Warning: Results May Come Fast

So knew that he had a gift for chess, but also understood that he wasn't maximizing his time—and screens were one of his biggest obstacles. He decided that in order to eliminate distractions he would have to remove internet service from his dorm room. This meant that to complete his coursework and use the internet, he'd have to leave the comfort of his room and go to the nearby library.

By removing the temptation of going online from his room, he also removed distraction from where he lived. He then started a ritual where he would turn off his phone and computer in his room and spend anywhere from three to four hours, undistracted, studying chess.

When I asked So what these sessions looked like, he explained that he would have a physical board in front of him as well as a paper by his side to jot down algebraic notation. As he would replay moves from his opponents' games, he would learn from them and then solidify new openings. He'd look to pinpoint his opponents' patterns and vulnerabilities, asking himself questions like: "What if they played this? Why didn't they play this?"

With his phone turned off and no Wi-Fi in the room, he was fully focused and engaged with no distractions.

As So was mastering his new training regimen, he appreciated the quote from NBA legend Kevin Durant, "Hard work beats talent when talent fails to work hard."

Like Durant, So knew he had the talent, it was just a matter of finding a training method that clicked.

In his dorm room in St. Louis, he found it.

"For most people, if they realize that the phone is a problem, they'd be very reluctant to put their phone down," said Ashwin Jayaram, So's roommate and chess teammate at Webster. "He was always able to have that discipline to just fully focus when he needed to work on his game."

Yasser Seirawan, a chess commentator and former top ten player, told me that while So learned to play chess in the Philippines, he became an exceptional professional player in the United States.

"He is an extraordinarily well-prepared, classical fighter," Seirawan told me. "He knows himself extraordinarily well. His strengths are very, very clear."

Before long, So was ranked number ten in the world. Then, in the fall of 2014 he won the Millionaire Chess Open, a tournament in Las Vegas, Nevada, that came with a $100,000 prize. So decided he would leave college and turn professional shortly afterward.

Unlike many of his peers who stream and have developed strong social media followings to supplement their careers, So went in the opposite direction. Seeing how positively turning off his phone had affected his practice routine, he yearned for that focused feeling all the time.

In early 2015, several months after leaving Webster, he decided to turn off his phone permanently.

. . . . .

So described the experience of turning off his phone as natural.

"I personally didn't feel any loss when losing my phone . . . I just felt much better. I had a lot more time," he told me.

So's level of focus improved further with practice. At his suburban home outside of Minneapolis, So can now work deeply for three hours, take a short break, and then pick up where he left off. On an average day, he puts in at least six hours of deep, undistracted work.

He uses a chess clock to track his progress. "I find that when you time your work . . . it's better."

What started out as a test at Webster to improve his game has become a hallmark of how So is able to compete at the highest level.

"I've been through so many failures in the way that I train in chess that when I find a good one, I tend to stick to it, like it's my treasure," he explained.

It's fair to wonder how a young professional in his twenties turns off his phone for good. The answer, So revealed to me, is that he has a strong support system. His adoptive mother, Lotis, who doesn't own a cell phone either, manages So's contracts and travel logistics. His sister, who does own a smartphone, helps manage his business affairs.

But So remains connected. He competes in online tournaments from his computer throughout the year as hundreds of thousands of fans stream and watch his every move. He also uses a computer to analyze games, with a chess engine that can tell him what works and what does not.

Not having a phone has also meant So has more interactions with people in person, which he prefers. He enjoys watching movies, streaming shows, reading books, going for walks, and swimming in his spare time. He is also a deeply spiritual person—in post-match interviews, he credits a higher power for all the good in his life.

As for social media, So tried having a Twitter feed that he maintained from his computer, but he ended it in 2023 after keeping it going for about a year. He also has not been active on Facebook since 2022. Why? So said he would spend a couple of hours every day on social media—and found it a waste of time.

As I put to just about everyone I spoke with for this book, I asked So whether he ever felt burned by not having a phone, especially as someone who travels all over the world and is highly sought-after by chess media and fans.

With a smile on his face, So told me that something came up recently: He wanted to show someone photos of two kittens he'd recently adopted. He said he has lots of photos of them on his iPad, but since he didn't have it with him, he wasn't able to show them off.

. . . . .

Back in Toronto, So was not able to defeat Carlsen. However, his second-place finish earned him $100,000 to cap off a successful 2023 season.

When I spoke with him several weeks afterward, he acknowledged that living without a cell phone won't necessarily work for everyone. But he said he was a happier person without one. As for his chess: "I just love the game. I love the career that I have. I love working on chess. And when I play beautiful chess, it makes me happy."

A LESSON ON FOCUS FROM ALEXANDER GRAHAM BELL

Wesley So's ability to maintain focus for long periods of time to advance his skills represents an important strategy: Working deeply without distraction will further your career.

After finding himself in a new country and in a college environment, it would have been easy for So to fall back on the old habits he'd developed living on his own in Manila. But he realized that to further his career, with smartphones all around him, he would need to eliminate distraction and focus. The idea of getting away from our phones to eliminate distraction isn't new, however—it actually dates back to the phone's inception.

In Robert V. Bruce's biography, *Bell: Alexander Graham Bell and the Conquest of Solitude*, Bruce details Bell's setup at his home at 1331 Connecticut Avenue in Washington, DC. Wanting to achieve focus and to eliminate distractions, Bell refused to have a telephone in his private study. He then took things a step further and required that anyone in his house who would accept a phone call couldn't do it within earshot of his work.

"I have found by experience that I can only deal with one thing at a time," Bell wrote in 1885. "My mind concentrates itself on the subject that happens to occupy it and then all things else in the Universe—including father, mother, wife, children, *life itself*, become for the time being of secondary importance."

If the phone did interrupt his work, he would joke, "Why did I ever invent the telephone?"

Newspaper reporters at the time reported that Bell banished the phone from his house. Bell was amused by this and would often repeat the claim.

· · · · ·

After Bell passed away, his wife, Mabel, refuted the claim that he disliked the telephone, and provided greater context.

"Of course, he [Bell] never had one in his study. That was where he went when he wanted to be alone with his thoughts and his work. The telephone, of course, means intrusion by the outside world." She added, "There are few private houses more completely equipped with telephones than ours at 1331 Connecticut Avenue, and there was nothing that Mr. Bell was more particular about than our telephone service here. For nearly all of the thirty-five years we have been here he saw personally to its proper working."

Bell was recognized as a scientist, innovator, and world figure. Often sought out by reporters, Bell's life was in the spotlight.

Yet Bell preferred to spend time alone, deep in thought.

He recognized that even his own invention in its most nascent form—something that could only make and receive calls—could rob his focus.

Why Deep Work Matters

Stefan van der Stigchel is a professor of psychology at Utrecht University in the Netherlands who specializes in the science of concentration and attention. Van der Stigchel describes the act of concentration as working like a muscle.

Similar to the process of building muscle in your biceps or calves through physical training, enhancing your ability to concentrate requires intentional and consistent practice. So, if you want to increase your ability to focus for extended periods of time, you have to train.

Van der Stigchel explains that removing a smartphone from the environment is a prerequisite for achieving deep focus. He compares leaving a smartphone nearby to someone on a diet trying to concentrate with a bag of cookies next to their laptop.

"At the end of the day, all of the cookies will be gone because you have a short moment of lack of conscious power, willpower, and you start eating," he said.

The skill to work and focus deeply is also the cornerstone of bestselling author Cal Newport's book *Deep Work*. He defines "deep work" as follows:

Professional activities performed in a state of distraction-free concentration that push your cognitive capabilities to their limit. These efforts create new value, improve your skill, and are hard to replicate.

In knowledge work, we have grown accustomed to constant interruption. Sometimes the break in focus can be caused by an incoming Slack message or an alert on your phone of an incoming email, text, or calendar reminder. Whatever the interruption is, we are living in a state of constant distraction.

Before I went through my own smartphone reset, I would finish a day of work and realize that all I had done was attend meetings and send emails. That is what my definition of productivity had become. But by turning off my phone, closing out email, and scheduling deep work blocks in my calendar, I was able to achieve focus. With that came a greater satisfaction with the work I was doing.

Newport found that the ability to do deep work was rare. After all, working deeply is hard; shallow work is easier. Therefore, your ability to work deeply comes with tremendous value and has the potential to take your career to the next level. But the ability to work deeply takes practice.

For Wesley So, being able to focus for several hours a day didn't come naturally at first. He started off in his dorm at Webster doing three to four hours of deep work each day. Today, So can work late into the evening, amassing as much as eight hours of deep work a day. He takes breaks—he might go for a walk or swim—but his ability to cultivate a life of working deeply took practice.

As hard as it may sound at first, you too can be like Wesley So. Perhaps you won't be solving chess equations, but imagine if you had uninterrupted time to focus on writing code, solving a proof, developing a legal case, or writing a novel.

Now you might be thinking to yourself, yes, not being addicted to my phone could very well help further my career.

But what about someone who needs a phone for work to succeed? What if you are an electrician who is constantly getting house calls? Or what if you are an on-call doctor and you need to respond to an emergency at a moment's notice?

Behold the Power of Workarounds

Dr. Scott Mittman began his training as an anesthesiologist at the world-renowned Johns Hopkins Hospital in Baltimore in the 1990s. Mittman stayed at Hopkins after he completed his residency, working almost exclusively as a clinician caring for patients and mentoring residents.

Mittman spends much of his time in the operating room, assisting pregnant women going through labor and delivery and also performing nerve blocks. Working at one of the top hospitals in the country, the cases Mittman encounters can be quite complex and require him to maintain an even, measured hand.

Whether or not Mittman is physically in the office or at home, he often needs to be available at a moment's notice day or night. As an on-call doctor with decades of experience, Mittman has naturally seen communication patterns and methods change considerably over the years.

When he started out at Hopkins in the '90s, doctors and other hospital staff used pagers. Then the first iPhone came out and Mittman noticed many of his colleagues making the transition to a smartphone.

Even as most of his coworkers began using text more at work, Mittman, then in his forties, remained skeptical of the smartphone's value.

"I really didn't see any great extra utility to getting one, especially as I started to see how many people were often glued to the screens in an unhealthy way," he said.

Mittman stuck with his pager.

Like many other hospitals, Hopkins eventually began issuing work smartphones to providers in order to more easily access Epic, a widely used electronic medical record system.

Mittman explained that the hospital-issued smartphones are so limited in their capabilities that colleagues will exchange personal phone numbers at the beginning of a shift to more easily text-message throughout the day.

Even though he was issued a work smartphone and could use it on call away from the hospital, Mittman decided to hold on to his one-way pager, a preference the hospital supports.

"The pager has worked for me . . . and it hasn't failed me, so I continue to use it," he said.

When Mittman is ready to head home for the day, he leaves his work smartphone plugged in charging at the hospital and takes his pager home.

"I found that the combination of a pager and ready access to laptop and desktop computers at home and at work were always enough for me."

What makes Mittman's approach even more interesting is that he also resisted getting a personal cell phone for many years, until he realized that for things like banking and two-factor authentication, having a smartphone was helpful. But he keeps it at home and doesn't take it with him outside the house. He leaves it plugged in, as if it's a landline.

This means that whenever Mittman leaves the house he does not carry a phone at all.

"Sometimes the rationale for having it is, 'Oh, I'll need it in an emergency,' but the fact of the matter is emergencies are very rare and usually there's some way of communicating in an emergency," he said. "I think the boundaries that I've set for myself are quite effective at limiting its use."

Mittman argues that physical separation from the smartphone is key to developing a healthy relationship with the device.

When he runs from his home in East Baltimore to the hospital each morning, the smartphone stays at home. When he goes out to the grocery store, the same.

Mittman talked me through a hypothetical emergency and how he would approach it. What would happen if his car broke down on the highway?

"I'd just walk along the highway and get off the first off-ramp. I'm not a worrier," he said, smiling.

Although Mittman suggests he might be the topic of countless jokes at work because he still uses a pager and doesn't carry a personal cell phone, when I spoke with two of Mittman's colleagues, they said he is beloved in the department, and is known for always being responsive.

And though he doesn't preach to colleagues, Mittman thinks it'd be worthwhile for physicians to spend less time on their phones at work *and* outside of the office.

"If you just leave your cell phone alone at least for several hours a day, I think people would find that they don't really need it as much as they think they do."

(According to Spok, the nation's leading paging company, there are at least 800,000 pagers in use around the United States.)

. . . . .

Establish an Emergency Valve

By turning off your smartphone, it's possible you'll get pushback from family and friends. The notion that you won't always be available to respond to messages immediately might bother some of them.

Before, when you had your smartphone on, there was an expectation that if you received a WhatsApp message, you would see it and respond immediately. And if a family member texted you and you didn't text back right away, you would likely hear about it.

These feelings from family and friends are natural. The problem is we have built communication habits that are untenable, as if we have all become on-call doctors and are expected to respond as quickly as possible whenever a new message arrives. So, before going through your detox you should create an emergency valve among family and friends.

What do I mean by an emergency valve?

Tell people how to reach you if there is an emergency. If someone is local, tell them they can knock on your front door if something pressing arises. If someone isn't local, tell them they can send you an email or call your work line.

Will anyone knock on your front door or call you at work? Probably not.

In most cases, people won't follow through, because in practice most people don't experience many actual emergencies. But you are at least giving people the option, and thereby recognizing that your detox could be an inconvenience.

If it makes it easier to establish your emergency valve, you can blame me as an opener. Tell people that you just read

Richard Simon's *Unplug*, were inspired by all the success stories, and felt empowered to live a deeper, more intentional life by turning off your phone.

It is also important to not take criticism to your detox personally.

Jose Briones (see page 197) broke up with his smartphone in 2019, opting instead for a Light Phone. He said he heard from friends about how he wasn't responding to messages on WhatsApp or other services. Briones didn't mind though.

"Your friends, if they are truly invested in your life, should be able to adapt if that means your life will be happier and that you are going to live a more fulfilled life," he told me. "So you need to advocate for that and come to understand that if somebody's unwilling to meet with you because you don't have blue bubbles, what does that really say about your friendship with them? If you don't have WhatsApp and they don't communicate with you . . . what does that say about that relationship as well?"

Relationship Investment

San Francisco is widely considered a center of the technology world. With the largest concentration of tech firms in the nation, the Bay Area has attracted top-tier talent from around the globe to companies like Apple, Google, Meta, and Uber.

Alex Hollender, a twenty-five-year-old user experience (UX) designer, was one of many East Coast transplants who came to call San Francisco home after graduating from college. Each workday, Hollender would walk the twenty minutes from his home in Potrero Hill to South of Market for work at an "ed tech," or education technology company. One morning in the winter of 2016, Hollender was halfway to his office and suddenly stopped dead in his tracks. He was listening to music on his iPhone with his headphones in his ears when a weird, uneasy feeling came over him.

Hollender couldn't remember putting his headphones on and pressing play.

At a standstill, he focused, trying to remember whether he put his headphones on after he closed the door to his house, or right before.

"They had just grown a life of their own or something and just found their way into my head every morning," he recalled.

As unsettling as the moment was, Hollender actually knew that his use of technology had been an area of growing concern for years.

Being Present Is Cool

When he was a student at Swarthmore College just outside of Philadelphia, Hollender recognized that he was spending too much time on Facebook, that he was unable to regulate his intake and also his emotions as he bounced from profile to profile.

"I was spending real amounts of time and emotional energy engaged with people or situations that I was learning about through Facebook that were not really part of my daily reality," he told me.

Things reached a breaking point after a gathering during Parents Weekend, where Hollender met the sister of a friend at Swarthmore. They friended each other on Facebook soon after, becoming "pen pals." Hollender felt it might lead to a relationship. He followed her activities on the platform, seeing updates she would post, as well as photos in which she was tagged.

Then, out of the blue, she pulled away. She told him that it was nice chatting, but that she wasn't interested any more. At that moment Hollender came to the realization that the relationships he was investing his time and energy in online were different from those in the physical world—they were easy to misjudge or simply misunderstand.

Miffed by the experience, he shut down his Facebook account.

Fast-forward six years. Hollender took off his headphones on his walk to the office and thought to himself, "Whoa, okay, this is starting to feel weird again. I'm doing things that I'm not really fully conscious of or not really entirely in control of."

Over the coming weeks, he thought about how unhappy his smartphone was making him. Living in San Francisco where most people were plugged in during and after work hours, Hollender had a front-row seat to the hyperactive hive mind that life there had become.

"One of the things I started thinking about pretty early on was this kind of urgency game that a lot of us seemed to be playing in San Francisco at that time," he explained.

Many of his colleagues and friends working in technology wanted immediate access to the internet, email, and messaging apps like Slack. There was an expectation that if someone sent you an email or text message, you would fire back a response as soon as possible. But this reality of everyone being on call by way of their phones didn't mesh with Hollender's outlook.

"I started thinking about it more and I realized that I don't think I'd actually received an urgent email or an urgent phone call in I don't know how long . . . nothing that was like, 'Oh my gosh, I have to put down what I'm doing,' and if I saw this email four hours later than seeing it right now, there would actually be a substantially different outcome."

"The need is kind of imagined," he continued, "or invented, and maybe it's invented as an excuse to justify using the device a lot, or I was thinking about it more at the time as, like, yeah, this kind of social status game that people were playing about how busy they were and how important they were."

One of the final straws for Hollender and his smartphone involved a relationship with a woman in San Francisco. They had a romantic history dating back to when they knew each other years earlier on the East Coast. One day they got into a disagreement over text and the exchange became, as Hollender described it, "really nasty."

"That really left an impression on me," he said. "Because too many times in my life . . . I had gotten into fights with people over text message and that damaged relationships. . . . You're typing so quickly and saying so many different things and not taking time to think about it."

Hollender wanted a life where there was more face-to-face interaction, conversations rather than mere connection. He was ready to simplify his phone setup. After doing some research, he called the Verizon store and switched to a basic phone.

When he told family and close friends about his decision, he faced some resistance, especially from his mom, who was worried she wouldn't be able to get in touch with him as easily, in what Hollender believed was a concern for his safety.

His counterargument: "Psychologically and emotionally, I didn't feel safe and secure," he told me. "I felt much safer with not having it."

When he switched to a basic phone, the most immediate benefit he found was in the area of life that was hurting him most: relationships. Because of how challenging it was to type on, he started to call people, something he had ceased doing with his smartphone.

Switching to a basic phone also gave him additional time to think before he responded to a text. He described his typical communications with people via smartphone as mindless. Whenever a thought began to form, he would immediately send it out over text. But when he switched to a basic phone, he became more intentional. And he also felt the need to communicate less frequently.

"It opened up more space for me to think . . . what do I like about this relationship? What do I get out of this relationship?"

He also noticed that because he was getting fewer alerts on his phone, he did not feel the same need to pull it out. When he was using a smartphone, whenever he would get pinged with a new email, an incoming transaction on Venmo, or a breaking news story, he would want to use his phone. "And so, the more I was on the phone, the more I was sending text messages out."

Even with the switch to a basic phone, Hollender felt that he was still very social, and that he had the same level of activity with friends—even though his frequency of communication decreased to one or two phone calls and text messages a day on average.

One of the unanticipated benefits of simplifying his phone was that, whenever he pulled it out in social situations, it was an easy conversation starter, as the novelty instantly drew people's attention.

"I would just know immediately that if I opened the thing up anywhere . . . someone would say something, and they always did. And I enjoyed that."

Hollender recalled being in Vermont at a café where he saw a woman with a basic phone on the table in front of her. He walked over and started chatting with her about her phone, and then took out his.

They became friends.

A daily ritual Hollender began was keeping paper charts on his bedroom door that listed key habits he was looking to improve. These included what time he went to bed, what he was doing socially, and what he was reading. By using paper instead of a digital tool, Hollender created a system to track his efforts by opening his door, rather than using a screen.

Reflecting on his decision to embrace a more analog existence, Hollender was amazed that he was able to slow life down.

"I can take some time, I can think, I can feel, I can just let time pass, which I think is such an amazing worker of miracles."

IS IT CONVERSATION OR CONNECTION?

The ability to have meaningful conversations with family and friends has no doubt suffered with the meteoric rise of the smartphone. As Hollender and so many others have experienced, a lot can get lost over text messages.

In her book *Reclaiming Conversation*, MIT professor Sherry Turkle argues that with digital communication, we are moving away from conversation, and are instead embracing "mere connection." And most people can't tell the difference between the two.

Here's the difference, according to Dr. Turkle:

Connection is when you apologize to your parents over text that you aren't able to come to a family meal.

Conversation is getting on the phone to apologize, and then hearing from your mom how hard she worked on the meal and how much you will be missed.

Connection is writing a text to a romantic interest and having your friends review it so that it's written out just perfectly.

Conversation is showing the real you to your partner, opening your heart with your words and body language.

We avoid face-to-face interactions to prevent difficult conversations, but how much stress does it cause the other party if we send a text that oftentimes gets misunderstood?

When we want to apologize to a friend, we might send a photo with an emoji. But by apologizing to someone in person, you have the power to exhibit empathy.

As an introvert, not having a smartphone forced me to get out of my comfort zone and connect with people on a deeper level with actual conversation.

And as Turkle explains, face-to-face conversation teaches us patience and allows us to connect on a deeper level with those whom we care about most.

Fewer Friends, Greater Depth

Saul Pwanson, forty-two, never considered himself to be a heavy smartphone user. There were certain games he played a lot and apps he checked throughout the day, but his discomfort with his phone largely had to do with privacy concerns.

When he realized in 2019 that his iPhone 4S had stopped working, he had to decide what phone he would get next. A software engineer based in Seattle, Pwanson explored alternative smartphone options and preordered a Purism Librem, featuring an open-source operating system not based on Android or iOS.

In the interim, since the phone wasn't ready to ship, he purchased an Alcatel Go Flip for $85 on eBay.

When Pwanson made the switch to the basic phone, many of his friends discovered that he wasn't responding to texts as quickly because of how difficult it was to type on the interface. What Pwanson realized was that many of the relationships he had over text weren't that strong at all.

"When text was taken away, I didn't want to see them and they didn't want to see me," he told me. "And so, the ones I did want to see, we carved out the space and we had much more focused and meaningful engagement, as opposed to a text here and there. And so I think I have fewer relationships, but the ones that I do have are a lot stronger or meaningful."

In August 2020, while the coronavirus pandemic raged, Pwanson left his job and was getting even less socialization. With many of his relationships reset from having his basic phone, Pwanson made a concerted effort to start blocking time off in his calendar for video conversations with friends. He tried to have at least one a day.

"Those conversations were deeply meaningful and I have several much deeper friendships, people that I hadn't even talked to much at all before that," he said.

Pwanson suspects that if he was using a smartphone at the time, he may have stuck with low-effort communication like texting.

"I may have been able to cling to the low-quality connections that I was having over text, feeling more like I was getting little dribs and drabs of socialization, but not having a smartphone forced me to dive in," he said.

The Purism phone that Pwanson ordered experienced significant delays, so his detox with the flip phone ended up lasting approximately two years. So when his Alcatel stopped working and he saw a promotion for a free Samsung Galaxy phone, he decided to reintroduce a smartphone to his life. But he made sure to not install mobile games or social media apps to ensure that he would use it for the "barest minimum of things."

Because of the detox, he said that he usually leaves his phone in his backpack, and it can stay there for days at a time. He explained that more often than not it will run out of battery, and then when a friend reaches out to ask him where he's been, he'll respond: "Oh sorry, it's been out of my line of sight for two days. I didn't notice."

"I use it when I need to do a specific thing and that's it," he told me, crediting the detox for rewiring his habits.

Pwanson told me he still has to put in the effort to be deliberate with his smartphone use. An example he gave was in the bathroom. There are studies that say as many as 88 percent of Americans bring their phones into the bathroom, and Pwanson wanted to take a stand against the practice.

Pwanson now uses his phone for common things such as GPS, short texts to arrange social plans, and dual-factor authentication for signing in to work projects. He told me bringing the smartphone back hasn't been perfect and that he sometimes spends too much time scrolling Reddit. "It's almost like I want something in that junk food category in my brain. Even though I've taken the worst of it out . . . I still find myself falling victim to it . . . I haven't weaned myself off of that dopamine circuit completely."

Pwanson started swing dancing in 2023, which was a great way to meet people in the community. He'll send a few text messages back and forth with friends to determine who's going to be dancing that week, but the longer conversations happen in person, which is how he prefers it.

Quality over Quantity

Like Pwanson's, many of my relationships suffered from a reliance on texting.

I had a few dozen friends I would text with throughout the year, but most of the exchanges were short and fairly shallow.

When I turned off my smartphone, to preserve the relationships I held dearest, I had to put in the effort to call people to make plans. As an introvert, this was uncomfortable for me, but I became much closer to my dearest friends. We'll still talk on the phone every month or two for several hours, which I prefer over a string of texts throughout the year. Without texting in the mix, another friend and I carved out time to be together in person once a week.

By rewriting your relationship with your phone, including a full breakup, you will inevitably lose touch with some people you might have been texting with as a primary form of communication.

But consider what you might gain: more time to spend focused, undistracted time with your closest friends. Plus, you'll have the clarity to invest in the relationships that matter to you most.

And that includes family.

Your Family Will Thank You

Attention deficit hyperactivity disorder, or ADHD, is a brain disorder most often diagnosed in childhood.

For Eoin O'Carroll, diagnosis came at the age of forty-five during the early months of the pandemic. Living in Amherst, Massachusetts, with his wife and two kids, O'Carroll realized that his executive functioning had degraded. The cognitive load associated with the pandemic, along with working from home with kids aged ten and five, put a level of pressure on O'Carroll with which he really struggled. With a constant flow of e-mails, slack messages, calendar appointments and alerts, O'Carroll felt he couldn't keep up.

"My brain was just not working at all," he told me.

As a technology reporter at the *Christian Science Monitor*, O'Carroll was well aware of the problems that come with smartphone overuse—and he knew that he wasn't immune to them himself. Some days he would scroll Twitter or Reddit far longer than he anticipated, spending time he wished he was investing in other places.

Eventually, the scrolling crept into time he wanted to spend with his family.

During dinner, he would check Wikipedia on his phone if he wanted to look something up, or the news when he was with his kids. It didn't mean O'Carroll was a bad father; he just wasn't present the way he wanted to be.

He tried different tactics recommended by experts to lessen the addictive aspects of his phone. He wrapped a rubber band around it to make himself more conscientious about using it. He made the phone less visually appealing by setting the color palette to grayscale. He changed his wallpaper to solid black.

None of it worked.

"Having my phone look less like a Montessori classroom and more like a Soviet apartment block would, I thought, make using my phone less tempting," he stated. "But instead it just made it less pleasant."

He continued, "This decoupling of 'tempting' and 'pleasant'—a defining feature of addiction if there ever was one—revealed to me that my problem was way bigger than I had thought. Fiddling with the display settings wasn't going to cut it."

O'Carroll decided that the best way to simplify his life was to not use his smartphone at all, so he switched his SIM card to an Alcatel flip phone and plugged his iPhone into his living room speakers, turning it into a dedicated MP3 player. When he made the switch, one of the immediate benefits was carving out time during the day to be with his wife and kids away from screens.

"I think what the biggest thing this change for me did was it created this barrier where I actually do now go on and offline," he said.

If one of his kids asked him a question about the Ninja Turtles, he fought his reporter instinct, and learned to accept that answers didn't have to come immediately.

"There is kind of this wall of separation there that had been worn down by the smartphone that's now back up. And so, when I'm with my family and when I'm playing with my kids, I'm usually on the other side of that."

What O'Carroll discovered is that when you realize your phone is taking you away from your family, you need to accept that change is necessary.

As Dr. Sherry Turkle writes, "Accept your vulnerability. Remove the temptation."

Moving away from texting improved the communication between me and my wife. Rather than texting throughout the day, we look forward to speaking to each other in the evening when we are together, from deeper philosophical questions to more mundane administrative household tasks.

We've also found that it benefits our kids. They can see and hear us talking to each other. Our loving comments register with them, as do our disagreements and how we resolve them.

"In families, the flight from conversation adds up to a crisis in mentorship," writes Turkle. "We need family conversations because of the work they do—beginning with what they teach children about themselves and how to get along with other people."

It might seem like a small thing, but writing down a shopping list will change the way you experience the grocery store. The process of texting with a family member or friend to check which bread to get, or whether a soup has too much sodium, makes the task more stressful and anxiety inducing.

If you live with someone, work on the shopping list together before you leave the house so you can be aligned on the purchases you plan to make.

Are there times my wife or I will come back from the store and there's something we missed? Sure. But it rarely happens, and our overall shopping experience has improved.

Nonscreen Activities for the Win

Cucumbers, zucchini, butternut squash, peppers, tomatoes, watermelon, peaches, and cherries. At first glance, it reads like a shopping list for the produce section. But tucked away outside of downtown South Bend, Indiana, you'll find all of these fruits and vegetables in the organic garden of Molly and Joe Gettinger.

From May to mid-October, after a long workday, Molly, a graphic designer, and Joe, a data analyst, are out in their front-yard garden with their three kids, all under the age of nine. Molly might be tending to the cucumber plants, which can produce as many as twenty a day, while the kids are under one of their peach trees, pruning or plucking off some of the sweet, succulent fruit.

The Gettingers spend hours each week on their garden, something they started in 2016, but there is one piece of technology that is always absent during the activity: a smartphone.

. . . . .

When Molly Gettinger reached high school in Kalamazoo, Michigan, her parents told her that if she wanted a cell phone, she would have to buy one herself. As one of the few kids without a phone, she found it awkward and challenging to make new connections with friends. She often felt like the world was moving in one way while she was moving in another.

"That experience is still with me," she told me, explaining that it left a lasting impact.

The feeling of being different stayed with Gettinger as she started at Holy Cross College at Notre Dame, Indiana, in 2009. She remembered walking into the Residence Life director's office and asking for a landline in her dorm room, one of only a few students who did.

Over time, Gettinger's decision to not get a cell phone became less about the financial side of buying one, and became more intertwined with her identity.

"It became part of who I was," she stated. "I wanted to be the person who was present . . . and who found other ways to communicate."

After graduating in 2013, she began working at a nonprofit in South Bend that required her to travel. For emergency reasons, she bought her first basic phone and used it for about five years before ending up with a hand-me-down iPhone SE in 2018. With poor cell phone service in her neighborhood, she had to connect to the internet to make phone calls. So, she switched over to the smartphone.

After not having one for many years, she was confident that she could create a system that would allow her to live a balanced life.

Gettinger now leaves her phone on silent so she doesn't see or hear text messages come in throughout the day. She sets aside one time during the day, typically in the evening, to respond to messages. That means if a friend sends Gettinger a message at 10 a.m., she won't respond until the evening.

Gettinger told me that most of her family and friends are used to having to wait twenty-four hours for a response.

"That experience [when I was younger] of not being a part of a group or of a movement drives me to want to create that community and sense of belonging in little ways like being present with my kids and not taking my cell phone out if I go out with friends in the evening," she said.

Grow More Together

Because of how intentional Gettinger is with her smartphone, her kids don't see her on it very much. Which is just fine by her, because that allows her and her family to spend more time on the activity that connects them most: their garden. Whether it's picking up free compost from the City of South Bend or pruning their tomato plants, the Gettingers experience their garden together.

When they first purchased their house, they started off small by focusing on salsa and pizza-making ingredients such as basil, cilantro, tomatoes, and peppers. They also planted their first fruit trees.

They expanded the garden over time, venturing into other foods such as pie pumpkins and watermelon, the latter of which the kids love even though they don't grow particularly well.

Because they don't have a lot of space for their garden in the front yard—only 1,000 square feet—they have to be strategic in the way they grow. That means growing vertically, which gives them more space.

"We prune all of our plants to get them to trellis up high," she explains.

Planting vertically has allowed the Gettingers to yield a lot of produce. Some days, they will pick twenty cucumbers, with as many as thirty pie pumpkins on the vine.

The Gettingers are self-taught, learning through local extension programs like Purdue Extension and also emulating strategies from self-help videos on YouTube. Each year, they pick a new skill to learn. When we connected in the summer of 2023, they were trying to get better at growing peppers.

But really, it's all about the act of going outside and connecting with each other outdoors. This delivers a feeling of satisfaction Gettinger believes you can't get from a phone.

"There's a chemical reaction in your body and your brain from handling dirt and being in nature," she said, attributing the release of dopamine while gardening as a game changer.

The Gettingers cook many of the things they grow, but also give them away to the community, further connecting them to those whom they live near.

Each member of the family has a role. Their oldest likes to find produce that he can pick himself, especially sun sugar tomatoes. Their middle child likes to walk around the garden carrying her zucchini and watching her parents garden.

"We're present in doing this activity as a family because there's not a phone interrupting that process,"

Gettinger said. "We aren't stopping to check things. We aren't getting dings in our pockets . . . we're all present."

. . . . .

This idea of getting out of your house to do meaningful activities is a critical step in filling your time. Whether it's building a garden like Gettinger, joining a ballroom dance group as Saul Pwanson did, going camping in the mountains with a loved one like Kate Emmons, or volunteering for the fire department like Stephen Kurczy, occupying your time by getting out of the house and away from screens is essential.

For me, one of the activities I committed myself to during my detox was golf.

Playing with my phone off completely changed the experience for me. Since I don't use a golf cart and carry my own bag, the walk between each shot gave me time to stay in the moment. I also like to daydream, which is only made sweeter by the beautiful natural surroundings of a typical golf course.

I often play by myself, but when I go out with friends, I feel a much deeper connection. We talk between shots, about life or why we couldn't have hit the last shot a little better. There's no distractions, only us and the next shot.

Don't Substitute One Form of High Dopamine for Another

Less than three months into my yearlong detox, the coronavirus pandemic forced lockdowns worldwide. Suddenly working exclusively from home and spending more time in the house came with a host of challenges.

One of those challenges was that I ended up seeking out other high-dopamine activities that were massive time wasters, including streaming YouTube from my computer and refreshing my email inbox repeatedly. It came to feel like, even without my smartphone, I was getting into many of the bad habits I had before. And because I was spending more time at home, my laptop became a kind of crutch, a high-dopamine replacement for my smartphone. My brain's need for mindless high-dopamine experiences was going unfulfilled, and I was trying to fill that void.

Here's how I overcame both: For my email inbox, I set aside specific times during the day to check it. At the time, I did worry that this could cause issues with colleagues if I didn't check it frequently. But I quickly learned that as long as I responded to messages the day they were received, or the following morning at the latest, everything was okay.

As for YouTube, I only let myself watch it when I was working out on the elliptical. This meant that if I was going to watch videos, it had to be while I was exercising, which actually served as a key motivator.

As mental health experts told me, when you go through your detox, your mind will naturally seek out replacement sources of dopamine. **Counter that drive.** Dr. Anna Lembke told me that many of us have set times and routines when we use our smartphones; with it out of the picture, it can be so easy at those moments to find something else to crave.

"I think the key is making sure that we're cultivating other ways of recreating that don't involve the device. . . . It can be so alluring and tempting to just replace our smartphones with our laptops," said Lembke.

"People will find replacement sources of dopamine," said Dr. Clifford Sussman.

He has found with clients that when one source of dopamine is taken away it is natural to seek out other sources of dopamine.

"If you take away their video games and get them off their console, then they'll go to their smartphone. . . . Anything that gives them that sort of dopamine flow, they'll take," he said.

Read a book, go for a walk, knit, go to the movies with a friend, join a board game night.

Our brains are like little alarm clocks—we're used to doing these highly reinforcing activities and behaviors at certain times. For me, putting the kids to bed was always a signal to my brain that it was time to go to the laptop. When that time approached, I felt that craving.

"It's really important to schedule other things to do during those peak intensity times," Lembke told me.

For example, if you're eating dinner and are accustomed to using your phone at the table, you'll likely crave a high-dopamine replacement activity. During your detox, keep screens away from the table. If you eat by yourself, ritualize a reading practice. Read a book or magazine at the table. If you eat with family or friends, focus on the conversation. If, like me, you're accustomed to picking up your phone after you put your kids to sleep, start a ritual where you exercise right after, do laundry, or talk to a friend.

The Power of Nature

Sarah LePage was always skeptical about bringing a smartphone into her life.

LePage, who grew up in East Africa, got her first cell phone in 2008 during high school and had to share it with her older sister. In 2010, when she went to college in Tennessee, she got her own basic phone. But as she looked around, she saw a world that was quickly changing, with most of her classmates getting smartphones. After graduating, she worked in Egypt for several years teaching English, and though she was in a foreign country, she kept her basic phone.

When I asked how travel worked for her in unfamiliar places, she told me she was tempted to get a smartphone but relied often on paper maps. "They don't run out of batteries," she said with a smile.

Eventually, LePage and her husband would settle with their children outside of Chattanooga, Tennessee. She remained steadfast, and never purchased a smartphone.

"I don't think I am disciplined," she told me. "That's why I have this flip phone."

At thirty, with two young kids and a screen time–heavy remote job with a land conservation company, LePage seeks out activities that don't involve technology.

Located close to LePage's house is Lookout Mountain, which offers hiking trails and sweeping views of the area. The mountain's conservancy needed someone to volunteer as a beekeeper. Since

LePage had a passion for bees and had done some work with them in college, she decided to take several interns under her wing and start an apiary.

During the warmer months, she goes to the apiary at least once every week, but in the fall during harvest season, her time with the bees increases. She teaches the interns, who are high schoolers, about beekeeping and native vegetation restoration.

With the interns by her side, LePage teaches a French style of honey harvesting called Warré. She then takes out a luggage scale and weighs the hives to determine what each colony will need through the winter months. Once she gets the bees to depart the hives, which can take days, she and her interns go into a kitchen, cut the comb, smash it up, and strain it through a colander. After a couple of days, they then rinse the wax and bottle the honey.

The work requires focus and devotion.

"I can't watch a baby while I'm doing it," she explained. "As a mom, you're often multitasking . . . so it's nice to just do one thing, it means that I have to be totally free, which is a luxury for me as a mom to be able to focus."

LePage said it's fun to work with interns at the community garden. "You kind of make it like a party," she said. "You have a lot of people so that it goes quicker and you all get sticky and you have to clean. It's a big cleanup at the end and there's honey all over the floor no matter how hard you try."

The act of beekeeping is a sensory experience, so when LePage opens up a hive, the smell of honey, flowers, and wax is incredibly pleasing. The yellow and gold colors make patterns that LePage finds beautiful each time she encounters them.

When I asked her whether she ever brings her flip phone with her to the apiary, she said, "It's a little hard when you've got your hands full. You have a smoker and gloves on."

This aspect of being outside to focus on a craft, while also investing in the community, is something that can bring tremendous rewards to anyone's life.

"It's part of being human," LePage declared. "There's a reason why that kind of work is enjoyable on a small scale . . . it is very life-giving to me."

QUIT TIP 9   Embrace Music in a New Way

As we learned earlier in this chapter, Alex Hollender's life improved dramatically by switching to a basic phone. One aspect was his consumption of music. With his smartphone, Hollender would play music regularly—it was a default activity. Many times, he would forget he was even listening to it, leading to a more passive listening experience.

Seeking to reinvent how he engaged with music by switching to a basic phone, Hollender had to be more intentional when he listened. With no SIM card in his old smartphone, he would take it out in his room some evenings and have to actively choose what he wanted to listen to.

He remembered turning on his smartphone after days of it being off and not listening to any music. He recalled a simple walk to the grocery store as an "insanely energizing" experience.

"I put my headphones in and I put the music on, and I was like, I'm not making this up, I was literally dancing the whole way to the store," he told me. Because he'd been listening to music less, he had to proactively set aside time to listen versus mindlessly hitting Play the way he used to.

He started an evening ritual where he would turn on music in his bedroom and intentionally not do anything else but listen. Hollender described it as "getting this thing back that I lost."

"It sounds kind of cheesy or overly dramatic," he explained, "but it was really like getting to listen to music all over again."

For Major League Baseball player Nick Castellanos, his relationship with music changed when he switched to his basic phone. He started a ritual of listening to vinyl on his record player after games. He'd ignite his firepit and put on ambient classical music, which relaxed him. His preference was something with piano, played softly. The vibe would provide him with the right headspace to reflect.

His record player goes with him when he travels, and his wife brings her favorite records as well.

Personally, I use a device called Mighty, which is a screen-free music player smaller than an iPod that allows you to listen to music from Spotify and Apple Music without a smartphone. The tool's tagline is "Freedom from the phone."

Going through a phone breakup doesn't mean you have to give up listening to music. In fact, it's an opportunity to regain the lost art of listening to music.

More Than Just Walking

Market Street to Mission Bay in San Francisco. International Boulevard to Fruitvale Avenue in Oakland, California. Chelsea to Lincoln Center and Greenwich Village to the World Trade Center in New York City.

These are some of Stacy Torres's favorite walking routes in the two regions she calls home: the San Francisco Bay Area and New York City. Born in 1980 in New York City to a working-class family, much of Torres's decision-making around when to get a phone was driven by cost. She didn't have a lot of money as an undergraduate and graduate student, and buying a cell phone was enough of an expense for her to forgo one.

But when her father was diagnosed with a serious form of lung cancer in 2005, she got her first cell phone in 2006 to help coordinate appointments and care. Wary of getting a phone with a contract that would include a monthly bill, she purchased an inexpensive basic phone with a prepaid card at a Rite Aid pharmacy.

Torres would stick with the phone for the next eleven years.

"I guess poverty helped keep me going for a while with that brick phone, as I was just a struggling graduate student at the time," she said.

Eventually, the basic phone became cost prohibitive because of limits on how many minutes she could use. She could have bought a smartphone, but instead opted for a Cricket flip phone for $30/month in 2017. Inundated with emails from students in the large lecture classes she was teaching in upstate New York, the thought of having a phone in her pocket with email, the internet, and messaging a swipe away was overwhelming.

At the time, she was pushing herself to make more progress on her academic research and was wary of how much of a distraction a smartphone could be.

"I am vulnerable to boredom or wanting instant gratification or distraction like anybody. And if I had the internet in my pocket all the time, I just don't want to even know what my life would look like," she said.

Torres ultimately lost her father in 2021, around the same time she also got out of a toxic relationship. It was a very challenging time for her mental health, as she confronted "some deep, dark depression stuff."

One of the ways Torres was able to compartmentalize and process some of the complex thoughts racing through her mind was walking every day for miles. Whether it's just to the train station and then to her office at the University of California, San Francisco when she's in Oakland, or from her childhood home in Chelsea to her alma mater Fordham University when she's in New York, Torres said the time she spends on foot helps break her pattern of ruminating.

The walks also help her process life's challenges without the distraction of a phone.

"I walk everywhere," she said. "It's therapeutic in the sense that it gives me some time to process, 'What am I feeling now? How is it relating to the past?' It just always lifts me out of whatever kind of low mood I might be in."

She also uses the time to plan how she will teach an upcoming course or prepare for an important meeting. She used to carry an MP3 player on walks, but now prefers to go without listening to music and let her mind "go where it will."

She likes to stay away from work emails on weekends, but when she does respond to a thread from the comfort of her home, it is that much more freeing to step away from the computer afterward and go for a walk.

"I don't want to say walking is a fix for all the problems in the world, but I always benefit from taking a walk and getting out," she said.

A GOOD WALK, UNSPOILED

"Walking is holistic: Every aspect of it aids every aspect of one's being. Walking provides us with a multisensory reading of the world in all its shapes, forms, sounds, and feelings, for it uses the brain in multiple ways," writes Shane O'Mara in his book *In Praise of Walking: A New Scientific Exploration*.

O'Mara, a professor of experimental brain research at Trinity College in Dublin, Ireland, argues that one of the biggest benefits of walking beyond the physical is its ability to clear one's mind from the day-to-day challenges of life.

Erling Kagge, a Norwegian explorer, was the first person to complete on foot the Three Poles Challenge—the North Pole, the South Pole, and the summit of Mount Everest.

For all of his walking, from the extravagant to the mundane, there is one common denominator: inner silence.

"Walking and silence belong together," he writes in his book, *Walking: One Step at a Time*. "To put one foot in front of the other is one of the most important things we do."

Here's what distinguished people have said about walking:

"I think that I cannot preserve my health and spirits, unless I spend four hours a day at least—and it is commonly more than that—sauntering through the woods and over the hills and fields, absolutely free from all worldly engagements."

—Henry David Thoreau, *Walking*

"When I am traveling in a carriage, or walking after a good meal, or during the night when I cannot sleep; it is on such occasions that ideas flow best and most abundantly."

—Wolfgang Amadeus Mozart

"The object of walking is to relax the mind. You should therefore not permit yourself even to think while you walk. But divert your attention by the objects surrounding you. Walking is the best possible exercise. Habituate yourself to walk very far."

—Thomas Jefferson, to his nephew Peter Carr in 1785

Invest in Yourself

Wangari Stewart always thought of herself as a very active person. A busy mom of two living in her hometown of Nairobi, Kenya, she had a good job and a busy social life.

Then one day, she didn't feel like waking up.

Barely eating and experiencing severe fatigue, she knew something was wrong. She saw a nearby doctor who told her that she was healthy, but perhaps she had an iron deficiency. She began taking vitamin supplements, but still didn't feel like herself.

Another challenge was her ongoing divorce. In the midst of it, she was having trouble finding the right path professionally, which came with financial worries about how she would support her family. And then there was the coronavirus pandemic, which complicated just about everyone's life even further.

She ended up going to a therapist and filled out a questionnaire. The therapist reviewed her answers and delivered some surprising news: She was clinically depressed.

.....

Wangari spent the first nineteen years of her life in Nairobi before moving to Perth, Australia, in 2005 to earn a degree in software engineering. After graduating she stayed in Australia, worked several jobs in the technology and finance sectors, got married, and had two children, one in 2013 and her second in 2015. She then moved back to Nairobi in 2018 after the unexpected passing of her father, something Wangari described as a "huge shock."

Returning to Nairobi meant she could be closer to family, but the city Wangari left in 2005 was a much different place in 2018. The way people communicated had changed radically. Instead of calling someone to make plans, most conversations took place on WhatsApp. Stewart described the experience of chatting with people over WhatsApp as having "no boundaries."

"Someone will write you a really, really long post and you're like, 'this could have been a conversation.'"

Wangari said she would get added to new WhatsApp groups all the time. Even if someone died, you'd get added to a new group. It spilled over to the business world too, with organizations using WhatsApp for work.

She also had pain points with Instagram, an experience she described as one of logging on and scrolling through pictures and feeling unhealthy. "It's a simulated world where everyone shows this very happy picture of themselves and then you know in reality they're struggling in their jobs, they're not as happy as it appears. And I think that puts a lot of pressure on people," she said.

Wangari began to rethink the relationship with the one device that was enabling all of these tools: her smartphone.

Unburden Yourself of More Than Your Phone

When Wangari was diagnosed with clinical depression, something her therapist told her struck a chord. "She was helping me recognize that I'm going through a lot," she said.

Her kids started going to therapy sessions too, and the therapist reminded them how much Wangari was going through as well as how best to support her. To bolster her physical health, she found a nutritionist in the United Kingdom who did a hair analysis test and found that Wangari's vegan diet was not sustainable. She recommended bringing meat back into her meals and also provided suggestions for how to respond to stressful situations.

Wangari started to have more energy—and the people around her began to notice.

"I'd come to accept who I am, accept where I'm at in life," Wangari told me.

In 2021, Wangari dropped her smartphone on the ground, leaving a big crack across the screen. When she took the phone to get fixed, the price was too much for Wangari to stomach, so she went to another shop and bought a basic phone for $10.

The breaking of her smartphone might've led to her buying a basic phone, but she'd been thinking about making the switch for a long time.

"If it [had] never happened, I think I would have still gotten there," she told me. "I think the phone cracking just expedited that process."

Almost immediately after she switched phones, she began to experience the benefits. She slept better at night without her phone at her bedside as a distraction. She stopped looking at articles about how to be happy through a divorce. And she also got rid of WhatsApp, which would have been far more difficult to do if she still had her smartphone.

The upside: It allowed her to discover who her true friends were.

Wangari began investing more in the relationships that mattered to her most: those with her mom, siblings, partner, and several friends. She made the effort to call them, and they would reciprocate. For everyone else, Wangari found that she might hear from ten people throughout the year and get a random call if they needed something, but with everyone else she stopped communicating.

She began meeting up with a friend for walks in Karura Forest outside of Nairobi. Surrounded by huge eucalyptus trees, it became a favorite place for both of them to exercise and connect with each other and nature. Being there, with all technology absent, was a way to find some inner peace.

Wangari would also set aside time two to three days a week to sit by a river—just her, the birds, and the beauty. Often she would fall asleep; at other times she'd just listen to the calming sounds of moving water.

Even inclement weather wouldn't stop her from getting outside. On rainy days, Wangari felt gratitude, as she walked across soggy terrain.

"I like the feeling of walking in mud. It feels very therapeutic to me," she explained. "I think it comes back to this feeling that I want to feel grounded."

But no matter what her stresses were, from being a single mom to overthinking finances or raising her kids the right way, the time to think gave Wangari perspective.

As she lay by the stream, she would tell herself, "Just center yourself and be present, be the best person when you're with the kids, and things will work out."

Without the ability to distract herself with a screen, Wangari was forced to confront her own thoughts and emotions. As she explained, the moments helped her to "sit and think, be uncomfortable, feel all the emotions" and then come up with a plan for moving forward.

Wangari remembered her daughter noticing that she wasn't on her phone as much, and that made her feel that her relationship with her kids was strengthening.

"I'm more present," she said. "I am comparing myself less to other mothers."

Wangari ended up using her basic phone for about two years and then returned to a smartphone in 2023 for travel. She uses a banking app, Google Maps, and a meditation app, but has been intentional about not adding social media or email to her phone.

.....

Wangari's ability to look inward and give herself the time and space to compartmentalize her thoughts is something that has become increasingly challenging for most people. Dr. Anna Lembke explains that too often we're distracting ourselves with the powerful stimulus of the smartphone.

"We're essentially drowning out our own thoughts and emotions where we're constantly able to run away from who we are and what we're thinking and our own conscience," she said.

Dr. Lembke described the experience of looking inward as terrifying for some because it forces you to encounter feelings and thoughts from which you were protecting yourself.

For Wangari, understanding that her smartphone was keeping her from connecting with herself was an insight that can be difficult to reach, and harder still to implement. Her cracked screen was the impetus, but she'd wanted to recalibrate and invest more time

Embrace Boredom

Unlike our youngest two kids, our oldest had trouble napping in the crib, and would often fall asleep on me or my wife while we played music in the background.

I vividly remember naps that would go as long as two or three hours—as I scrolled on my phone the entire time.

During the winter months, he would wake up in a daze from an afternoon nap and I would look out the window: It would be dark out. I'd often think, "What did I do with myself the last two and a half hours?"

My eyes had lost the ability to stare, to think, to be bored.

Many of us think boredom is a bad thing, and when we sense it coming we quickly grab our smartphones to fill the void.

But we shouldn't.

"We have gotten to a terrible place where we are so averse to boredom that we cannot disconnect at any point," said Dr. Michael Rich, the director and founder of the Digital Wellness Lab at Boston Children's Hospital. "And I would argue that boredom is where creativity and imagination happen. . . . I mean, when was the last time you saw a kid lying on their back in the grass making shapes out of the clouds? You just don't do that anymore."

The newfound ability to embrace boredom was something that came across in so many of the people I interviewed, from Adam Weiss working in his chemistry lab (see page 43), to Josh Haskell (see page 71) staring at the wall in his dorm after a difficult conversation.

When you feel bored, stop, breathe, and embrace the moment.

in herself well before it happened. She just needed that final nudge.

With smartphones, Dr. Sherry Turkle has noted, we don't give ourselves moments for quiet. We don't allow ourselves the space to feel vulnerable. Instead, we try to fill those gaps with texts, scrolling, or the latest news item.

"One of the rewards of solitude is an increased capacity for self-reflection," she writes. "Solitude is important for everyone, including the most extroverted people. It's the time you become familiar and comfortable with yourself."

Before my own yearlong detox, I defined solitude as sitting on a lawn chair scrolling through my phone. Boy was I wrong.

"Eventually we learn a lot about ourselves and our conduct and our lives and we get perspective and we get meaning," said Dr. Lembke about the power of detox. "We'll have reconnected to ourselves."

CHAPTER 5

Reintegration

Your detox is complete. You have recalibrated your brain not to crave your smartphone. You have also restructured the way you live. But what happens if you decide to add a smartphone back into your life?

I first started interviewing people for this book in the fall of 2021, so for some, it had been more than two years between our initial interviews and my deadline to turn in the manuscript. And I had follow-up questions: Did most people turn their smartphones back on? Did their detoxes persist? What did their phone setups look like? I wanted to know what they had learned along the way.

Here's what I learned:

- Writer Kate Emmons (see page 79) continues to embrace the off-by-default philosophy. She switched to a basic phone, and only turns it on to make calls when she is traveling alone.

- Anthony Donataccio and Michele Perry (see page 121) are still using their basic phones, something Perry describes as a "blessing" for both of them.

- Stephen Kurczy (see page 95) still doesn't own a cell phone and said his students at Providence College think "I'm utterly insane."

- Lawyer Joe Pankowski (see page 87) continues to practice the off-by-default philosophy and still uses his phone for digital tickets for Florida State football games.

- Wangari Stewart (see page 176) started her own business and decided to reinstall WhatsApp on her phone to better engage with customers. In 2024, amid the upheaval in Nairobi where protesters stormed the country's parliament, Wangari said that because of her two-year detox, she felt in control of the time she spent on her smartphone, setting aside fifteen minutes each evening to see what was happening, and then putting it away.

In fact, most of the people I interviewed were still experiencing a reduction in screen time as a result of the detox.

But not everyone had held serve, so to speak. There were two follow-up interviews I conducted with Eoin O'Carroll (see page 157) and Alex Hollender (see page 146) that were eye-opening, informative, and might help guide your decision if and when you decide to use a smartphone again.

Because Life Happens

I first connected with Eoin O'Carroll in 2021, a year into his smartphone breakup.

At the time, he was connecting on a deeper level with family (see page 157), and his decreased dependence on his smartphone was helping him with his recent ADHD diagnosis. Fast-forward two years and I found myself reading a preview to his email that I wasn't expecting:

> *I'm worried that I might end up messing with your thesis at the eleventh hour.*

I opened it up and read on:

> *That's because not only have I gotten back together with my ex (now an iPhone 13 mini), but now I'm also wearing an Apple Watch. What's more, my two kids—ages eight and thirteen—now have three (!!!) smartphones between them.*

I was a little floored. But as I read on, everything started to make sense.

> *The turnabout came suddenly in September 2022, when my then seven-year-old son, Declan, was diagnosed with type 1 diabetes. Overnight, I had to learn how to be his pancreas, continuously*

monitoring his blood sugar, adding up grams of carbohydrates, and calculating the right insulin dosage every time he eats. As you can imagine, my flip phone was nowhere close to being up to the task.

Declan, for his part, carries two phones, an iPhone that links via Bluetooth to his wearable glucose monitor (a Dexcom G6) and a "personal diabetes manager"—basically an Android phone with specialized software—that controls his wearable insulin pump (an Omnipod 5). The iPhone has an app that shares his glucose concentration with me, my wife, his sister (who had been asking for an iPhone for the year leading up to his diagnosis), his grandmother, and his school nurses so that we can intervene when necessary.

I'll leave it to you to determine whether this counts as "coming full circle" or "eating crow." I suppose it depends on how strident I was when we last spoke!

O'Carroll and I connected on a video call the following week. As I dug deeper about his transition to a smartphone, I was amazed at how much he had learned from his detox, and how it informed his use of his smartphone currently.

In understanding his own struggle to achieve consistent focus with ADHD, when O'Carroll brought the smartphone back into his life after two years, he created a system that allowed him to maintain control over his phone, rather than the opposite.

He understood the pitfalls, recalling a period in his life when he would check his phone for the time and then, hours later, still be standing in the same spot scrolling on Wikipedia, reading about the French Revolution.

"What I really needed to do was figure out a way to get my smartphone to work with my ADHD," he said.

After some trial and error with different tools, O'Carroll discovered the Shortcuts app, a tool that allowed him to make his home screen a task board. When he showed me what it looked like, it reminded me of my Trello board for work (imagine a whiteboard with tasks arranged on sticky notes).

Task cards that O'Carroll had set up included Shop, Drive, Metabolize, Listen, To Do, and Connect. If he taps on Shop, his screen shifts to all of the tools he uses for online shopping. He also uses the Focus feature on his iPhone, allowing him to tune things out that don't matter and focus on what does.

But O'Carroll admits that he still looks at his phone too much.

That's why when he's with his family in person, he turns it off. Rather than having to hold down two buttons and then swipe to turn off, O'Carroll created a blue power button on his home screen that makes for a frictionless experience.

"By having the power button on the home screen, on the very first screen that I see, it alters the possibility. It's a bright blue button that says you can turn off your phone. And that's really powerful," he said.

When his daughter Ciara's school day ends one hour before he has to pick up his son Declan, the two of them spend quality time together. If the weather is nice, they'll go to a nearby park to throw a Frisbee together. If the weather is chilly, they'll go to Dunkin' Donuts or sit in the car and talk.

"This hour with Ciara is really, really important to me," he told me. "It's the one time built into each day that I can devote all of my attention to her. . . . Needless to say, my phone stays off during this time."

For O'Carroll, the smartphone has enhanced his family's life. It has shifted his son's diabetes diagnosis from "a crisis to being a nuisance," for which he is grateful.

By going through a two-year smartphone detox, O'Carroll learned how to use his smartphone intentionally when he brought it back into his life.

"It reset my relationship with mobile technology. Before it was not intentional. It was unstructured," he told me. "It made me realize that if we don't use technology intentionally . . . then what it really means is that it's structured by somebody else."

When a Lifeline Is More Important

Sarah Daniels is a child life specialist at St. Jude Children's Research Hospital, a pediatric treatment and research facility headquartered in Memphis, Tennessee, that focuses on pediatric diseases such as leukemia and cancer.

Daniels, who works primarily with young adults and teens in the hospital, has spent years researching how devices and social media interface during a patient's treatment. Much of the research on smartphones and social media for healthy young adults has centered on how dangerous they are. But when a cancer patient comes to the hospital, Daniels notes that it's a much different experience.

"They're separated from their peer groups, they're not going to school, they're not engaging in their sports anymore. So their social worlds are disrupted significantly at time of diagnosis," she said.

Which raises the question: Do screens exacerbate that stress?

Daniels has found that smartphones can be a "lifeline" for children during a difficult time in their lives. She explained that they can be used to help children cope and communicate with the outside world following a devastating diagnosis.

When patients come to the hospital, they're told when to take medicine, how often to come to the hospital, and what they can and can't do—leading to a diminished sense of independence.

"What's nice about the smartphone and social media is that's one area that they can exercise their control," she said. "They're already in this context that's very different than their peers, and if they can't maintain some of the normal social activities that their age group is participating in, it becomes more stressful for them."

If a smartphone helps connect you to the world during a difficult time, your well being takes priority.

BEING PRESENT WITH FAMILY

In a 2014 study, pediatrician Jenny Radesky wanted to gain a better understanding of how smartphone use impacts the relationships between caregivers and children.

Observing fifty-five caregivers eating with one or more young children at fast-food restaurants, Radesky and her researchers found that forty used devices during the meal, and a majority paid more attention to their phones than their children.

Radesky found that the kids who had parents that were most absorbed by their phones were the most likely to misbehave to get their parents' attention.

"These face-to-face interactions are the primary way that children learn," said Radesky in an NPR interview. "They learn language, they learn about their own emotions, and about how to regulate those emotions. They learn by watching us. . . ."

Obvious concerns surface when you read something like this. What must a child be thinking when a parent is paying more attention to a device than to them? Also, this study is now over a decade old. How much worse has it become?

"From infancy, the foundations for emotional stability and social fluency are developed when children make eye contact and interact with active, engaged faces," writes Dr. Sherry Turkle. "Infants deprived of eye contact and facing a parent's 'still face' become agitated, then withdrawn, then depressed."

School principal Seth Lavin (see page 62) gets to see the distracted state of parents firsthand.

"It is really sad, and I think it really challenges kids and put some tough stuff inside them that shows up in odd ways at school," he told me.

With the publication of Jonathan Haidt's 2024 book *The Anxious Generation*, throngs of parents are mobilizing to create clear standards around phone-free schools and limits for how early in life kids have access to smartphones.

I've been encouraged to see the overwhelming response to the book, but what do we do about our own behavior as adults?

The school we send our kids to has become phone-free. But when I see parents holding their kids' hands at pickup after school looking down at a screen, or looking down at their phones while their kids play in a school sporting event, I wonder what kind of message that sends.

If our kids see us addicted to a device, spending less time focusing on them and more time on a screen, will they take our warnings on the harm of too much screen time seriously?

Tread Carefully upon Reentry

Bringing a smartphone back into your world can be an incredibly slippery slope, but unique challenges and circumstances are part of life, and not having a smartphone long-term may not be realistic for some.

Do I still think that doing a smartphone detox for at least two months is necessary to reset your relationship with it? Absolutely. But I'm not an absolutist.

After your detox is complete, think critically about what you want your life to look like if you do decide to bring your phone back in. Dr. Michael Fraser, a screen addiction specialist, said that if someone decides to reintroduce a smartphone, they should first ask themselves what they learned from the detox process. That way, they can determine which things can be used on their smartphone to increase productivity, but not detract from other areas of life.

For many, including most of the people I interviewed, going back is not an alluring option. But if you feel you don't have a choice at this stage in your life—like Eoin O'Carroll—thoughtfully plan what your life will look like when you turn back on your smartphone.

When my yearlong detox was complete, I knew I didn't want to get rid of my smartphone entirely. There were, admittedly, certain aspects of it that I appreciated and missed. Those included GPS for longer drives or podcasts for monotonous tasks around the house. My phone will stay off for days at a time, but in those moments when I need it, I'm grateful I have it. However, I know that if I hadn't gone through a detox and experienced living without my smartphone for an extended period, it's unlikely I would have the discipline I maintain today.

. . . . .

When I first reached out to Alex Hollender in late 2021, he was living in Vermont, five years into his smartphone-free journey. He had moved away from text-based conversation and enhanced his ability to connect with people on a deeper level (see page 146).

When I contacted him two years later, he told me he'd moved to New York City and was using a smartphone again. His LG Exalt basic phone broke and when he couldn't get it repaired, he tried out a Nokia basic phone, which died as well. So he decided to go back to an iPhone.

How did his transition go after being off of a smartphone for seven years?

"I've just completely regressed . . . I still don't have social media or anything, but I'm looking at it a ton."

He downloaded dating apps, which led to some "pretty serious addictive behavior." He also is very interested in AI chatbots; whenever he's curious about a topic, he'll type a question into his phone in search of an immediate response. Hollender explained that reintroducing a smartphone meant that he started communicating more frequently. He also found that when he confronts challenges during his workday or is feeling lonely, he'll reach for his phone to fill that void by contacting someone. If he doesn't hear back from that person, he gets frustrated.

"Messier" was the adjective Hollender used to describe his new communication patterns. As a result, Hollender said he had recently purchased a new basic phone: a Kyocera Dura XV Extreme+. "I'm excited to switch back and re-embrace that," he declared.

As you'd expect, reintroducing a smartphone into your life will most likely come with challenges.

"For everybody who decides to go back to trying to use in moderation, it is a constant battle," said Dr. Lembke. "The battle itself, in my opinion, is for most people not worth the effort and very painful."

With your neural pathways reset, the idea of going back to a smartphone may be unappealing, which is why many opt for a more permanent solution, such as a basic phone or going off-by-default. Others may feel that they have the discipline to turn their smartphones back on and still control their usage. But proceed with caution.

As with anything addictive, returning to your smartphone can lead to many of the same bad habits you were experiencing before. Dr. Lembke believes that we actually have to separate ourselves from the devices.

"I had hoped for a long time that through various guardrails . . . that we both individually and collectively as a society could figure out a healthy relationship with the technology. But as time has gone on, I have become less and less optimistic about that," she said.

If you decide to bring a smartphone back into your life, consider using the off-by-default philosophy; it renders the phone more or less inert, powered off and powerless.

Regression

After your detox is complete, if you feel yourself regressing, consider doing another detox. Don't view it as a one-and-done deal.

Regression is natural, especially for a device as addictive as a smartphone. So, if you simplified your phone for your detox approach, try it again, or find one of the other three approaches that you think will set you up for success.

Dr. Hilarie Cash said dropping our guards after a detox is common, especially because of how alluring the smartphone is.

"It's a very tough struggle, and it's not a struggle anybody should be taking on alone," she said.

Just like I recommended before you started your first detox, ensuring you have a community of family and friends to support you through this process is critical.

Dr. Cash also recommends hiring a therapist who understands the problems that can develop with technology. A therapist will help with accountability as well as with adjustments to your detox depending on life circumstances.

Don't be discouraged. The many designers and engineers who created our smartphones designed the experience to be difficult to resist.

Don't let that stop you from being the best version of yourself.

CHAPTER 6

Helping Others Quit

"Do I want to live my life like this?"

That was the question Jose Briones kept asking himself. The twenty-four-year-old had recently completed his Master of Divinity degree from Andrews University in Michigan and was working as a minister for a network of churches in rural Georgia.

As invested as Briones was in the community-based work he was doing, he knew something was wrong. He was spending a lot of time internet scrolling, as well as creating content online and messaging on social media. In addition, his work involved traveling by car from one church to another, and he would mount his phone on his dashboard and stream Netflix.

Eventually, he decided to look at his phone to determine how much time he was spending on it. The number alarmed him. Thirteen hours.

More than half of each day was spent on his phone.

"I felt like my life was lived online most of the time," he admitted.

Briones wanted to live a more balanced life. With most of his waking hours spent on a screen, he needed to simplify things—and bought a Light Phone at the end of 2019.

"My main motivation was just that I wanted to spend more time with the people and things that I wanted to do, which was taking care of my health, taking care of my family, and taking care of my overall well-being," he said.

Briones quickly realized that he couldn't do much with his new phone. There were no easy shortcuts, which meant the amount of time he spent on his phone was immediately cut by more than half.

What did Briones do with the extra time? He spent it with his wife and friends, participated in book clubs, and found more time for walks with his dog. He felt greater focus in his work without the constant temptation of digital media. The process was so empowering that he started to document it, posting videos to YouTube about switching to a Light Phone.

Switching wasn't easy at first. In fact, at the beginning of the pandemic, Briones went back to using his smartphone for about a week. But when he reintroduced it after months of being away from it, he knew he couldn't go back for good. He told himself, "I don't want to waste my time in front of a screen for the rest of my life."

In addition to speaking about his experience with the Light Phone, Briones started to add additional videos to his YouTube channel reviewing other basic phones. Whether it was the Alcatel Go Flip 4, the Xiaomi Qin F2 Pro, or the Sonim XP5plus, Briones soon became the authoritative online voice for smartphone alternatives.

"I started making videos documenting my experience. And then people started to ask questions, and then I started to become more knowledgeable about those questions and about how to help people," he said.

As his YouTube channel grew in popularity, Briones launched a website with a Dumbphone Finder feature (https://dumbphones.pory.app/) that allows people to sort and learn about dozens of basic phone options on the market. There is a filtering function to see how many stars Briones has awarded to each phone, network availability, group text functionality, podcast/music options, and so forth.

"The goal is that people come [to my site or YouTube channel], find the device that they want, and never come back again," he explained. "I learned that it's better to give people value, and if they find a device that they love and that helps them . . . then my YouTube channel accomplished its mission."

Paying It Forward

You don't have to go to the lengths that Briones did, but after you've completed your smartphone detox, you'll likely want to tell others about your experience. It is something you should be proud of and embrace.

There's a good chance your friends, family, and coworkers want to spend less time on their phones, too. And because you now understand the impact a smartphone detox had on your life, you get how it can really help someone else.

"It's such a huge motivator for me," Briones said. "Somebody regained six hours of their life every single day so they can spend time with their family doing the things that they truly love and changing the way that the algorithm works for them."

Briones said he gets questions from viewers about everything from how he manages a QR code at a restaurant to purchasing tickets for concerts and sporting events with a basic phone.

"You have to learn to advocate for yourself," he said.

It can make you feel vulnerable not having the convenience that most of society takes for granted, but it's also okay to speak up. If you're trying to log in to a financial account and it requires two-factor authentication to verify, call up the company and tell them you don't have a smartphone and see what your options are. I've found that email can often be used as a substitute to send codes for login. If there are no physical menus at a restaurant, tell your server that you don't have a smartphone to scan a QR code and that you'd like a paper menu.

You Are Not a Stranger Here

As I started to open up to people about my smartphone philosophy, I found the topic elicited passionate responses. People wanted to know more—and were relieved that they weren't alone in struggling with their screen time.

You don't have to stand on the curb of a busy intersection waving a poster that says: "I unplugged!" But like Jose Briones, who decided he wanted to be a resource for people looking to choose simpler technology, you too can be a resource—even an inspiration—for family and friends to live a better life.

Dr. Marc Potenza, an addiction expert, argues that there's a stigma associated with addictive behaviors and that some people might not want to open up about their journeys. But with so many people struggling with their smartphone use all around us, Potenza sees this moment as an opportunity to show compassion, to let people know what a healthier relationship with our phones looks like.

"Part of breaking down the stigma is having people share their stories and be comfortable," he said.

Dr. Anna Lembke believes the same—when you tell someone that you don't have a smartphone or aren't easily reachable, people might think you are crazy. That's why, she argues, it's important "to destigmatize the detox and destigmatize not having a smartphone."

When Briones, who now lives in Colorado, attends Denver Nuggets basketball games at Ball Arena, he buys his tickets at home and prints out the receipt. He then brings the receipt with him to the arena and visits the ticket resolutions counter. After showing his ID and providing his email address, the Nuggets representative writes down his name and seat number on an official slip of paper and that allows him to go in.

"You have to be willing to be a little bit of a nuisance for the sake of living your values," he said.

Inspiring Others

Justine Haupt is a space engineer and astronomy researcher who lives on Long Island, New York.

Working with incredibly sophisticated technology as a researcher at the Brookhaven National Laboratory, Haupt is clearly someone who embraces technology and its potential. However, one piece of technology Haupt has resisted is a smartphone.

"I just never bought into the smartphone thing to begin with," she told me, explaining that she always saw it as an unhealthy addiction.

In her free time, Haupt develops her own inventions, what she described as open-source projects on which other researchers and engineers can collaborate. These include a paragliding motor, a system that endows a Chevy Bolt with self-driving capabilities, a large-format 3D printer, and a way to turn "your unwanted 35mm camera into an accent/spotlight for $10."

Her personal website offers instructions on how to build all of these things, giving people an opportunity to expand on her work. But there was one project that Haupt was working on that struck a chord. In 2020, Haupt posted pictures and the design files for a new mobile rotary phone.

When she updated her website with a description and pictures, she didn't think much of it, other than taking pride in what she had developed. But soon after, Haupt received a message from a friend saying that someone had posted her mobile rotary phone on Twitter and it was going viral.

Eventually, there was so much interest that Haupt's website crashed.

"They [the webmaster] thought I was having a distributed denial of service attack. I had to talk with the webmaster to say, 'Oh no, I think this is actually real.'"

Soon, *Wired* and other publications began reaching out to her to learn more about the device.

"I was surprised how much people resonated with it," she said.

Haupt called it the Rotary Un-Smartphone and gave it the tagline, "A cell *phone*. You know . . . for making CALLS."

The phone is pocket-sized, lightweight, and allows you to use your own SIM card. As interest for the phone rapidly increased, rather than just providing instructions for how to make it, Haupt decided to sell the parts herself.

Customers can either use the rotary dial to call someone or program numbers into the phone and use the speed dialing function. Available in five colors, the phone has basic text messaging, as well as a contact list.

Originally, Haupt thought the infatuation with the product had more to do with the novelty of how cool it looked. But she then started to hear from more and more people who were buying it as a way to reject smartphone culture.

"I had so many people saying, 'It's really time. I'm really ready to move on from my smartphone, but there isn't another compelling alternative that I've really wanted to adopt,'" she said.

Haupt encountered production roadblocks. With four custom-printed circuit boards, she admitted that it's incredibly complicated to make. Starting out in her mom's basement, she eventually found office space and brought on a business partner to help.

What started as a side project born of procrastination has now made Haupt realize how much people want autonomy over how they use personal technology.

"My hope is that anyone who chooses to use one of these, whether they build it themselves using the open-source documentation or just buy the kit, is doing so because they want more control over their technology," said Haupt.

You don't need to start a movement or invent an alternative to the smartphone to make a difference in other people's lives. So many people are struggling with how they use their smartphones that it's not hard to find folks who readily acknowledge it. So, after going through a detox and resetting your life, tell people about your journey. You might be surprised by the reactions.

Notre Dame student Josh Haskell (see page 71) talked openly with friends about his decision to switch to a basic phone. Soon, some of those friends were trying it. Eventually, he wrote a letter to the editor at the Notre Dame student newspaper that advocated for switching to a basic phone. It was one of the most-read articles of the year.

Joe Wakley, who went through his phone breakup alongside his girlfriend, Ella Jones (see page 112), also spoke openly about the process with friends. When he sees someone struggling with their phone use, he'll ask, "How do you feel about that?'

School principal Seth Lavin (see page 62), whose basic phone usually invites teasing and laughing from his students whenever he takes it out, also notes that it leads to conversations.

"They see me as sort of like a phone radical," he told me. "And that opens them up to talk about it. . . . It pushes them to think a little bit or create space for them to reckon with their own phone stuff."

But perhaps one of my favorite examples of helping others be in the moment is musician Jack White, who has used his fame and passion for living a cell phone–free life and created an experience at his concerts that is wholly unique: He doesn't let fans use cell phones at his shows.

Inspired by comedian Chris Rock, who also doesn't allow phones at his performances, White hired a company called Yondr, which provides smartphone pouches that magnetically lock inside a venue. Once someone leaves the venue, they can unlock their pouch and access their smartphone.

When fans go to a show where Jack White is performing, they're greeted by a sign that says, "Enjoy being phone-free."

White wasn't sure what the reaction would be to something so drastic. For example, would fans demand their money back if they couldn't use their phones? But White said fans embraced it.

"To my surprise, everyone loved it," he told the United Kingdom's Channel 4 in 2019.

He remembers sitting backstage after a sold-out show at a ten thousand–seat arena when his photographer opened up Twitter to see how many people had posted about the show, since everyone's phones were locked at the time.

"Five people tweeted about it," he said. "If everyone had their phones, maybe upward of ten thousand people would have tweeted about that moment."

Conclusion

Several weeks before I submitted the manuscript for this book, I checked back in with Major League Baseball player Nick Castellanos, whose cell phone journey opened the book.

Castellanos was in Clearwater, Florida, preparing for the upcoming 2024 season. A lot had happened to him since we'd last talked. After his breakout season with the Reds in 2021, he secured his largest contract as a player, a five-year, $100 million deal with the Philadelphia Phillies. He helped the team reach the World Series in 2022 and continued to produce afterward, earning his second All-Star Game selection in 2023. Castellanos also cemented his name in baseball history during the 2023 National League Division Series, becoming the first player to hit two home runs in back-to-back playoff games.

But when he and I talked, he was eager to chat about something else. After going through a smartphone detox for over a year, he told me that he had turned his iPhone back on.

The motivation was the birth of his second son, Otto. On the road, Castellanos wanted to be able to FaceTime for doctor's appointments and see his son before games.

He told me his iPhone looks completely different now than it did before his detox.

"Before I did my detox, I had six, seven pages of just apps, all different kinds of games, all different kinds of social media apps," he told me. "If you look at my iPhone now, it doesn't look like a normal iPhone. I don't have any apps or games. The only things that I have are things that are 100 percent necessary."

Castellanos told me that he installed two apps: Uber Eats for food deliveries and Teamworks, an app used by the Phillies organization to communicate with players.

After the detox, reintegrating the smartphone into his routine was simpler because his loved ones had grown accustomed to him not always responding immediately to messages, which he believes eased the transition.

"I'm still notorious for being terrible with my phone," he said. "I'll go through times or days where I'll just leave it and forget where I put it. Before I did the detox, my phone was fully charged every night next to me. I always knew where it was, but after that reset, my dependency on it has changed dramatically."

Castellanos had taken what he learned from his detox and mentored younger players on the Phillies.

"I can see how a lot of times their attention span will get taken away by what people are saying on Twitter, or who's popular, or projections, or what people think about them, the opinions of others, and it really takes them out of their everyday."

But what stuck out most to me in our conversation was that Castellanos was planning to "unplug" again, creating more separation between himself and his iPhone so that he doesn't have constant access to the internet. During his reintegration phase, even without addictive apps, Castellanos told me he's still susceptible to mindlessly watching videos or getting consumed by internet content.

Reflecting on the last three years, he said that if someone wants to be a master of their craft, turning off their smartphone is a good first step.

"I think that anybody in any profession, whether you're a doctor, a teacher, a scientist, or a professional athlete, can benefit from simplifying their lives," he stated. "Ideally, the goal is that you're disciplined enough to use an iPhone, and not have it use you."

. . . . .

When you first opened this book and read Castellanos's story, you might have had an inkling that turning your phone off could bring benefits to your life.

I hope you've seen that change is possible. That what might've begun as a hope that you could do this has turned into you *can* do this.

You could be from the heart of the rust belt like Adam Weiss, seeking to further your career as a scientist and deepen your relationships with friends. Or a writer like Kate Emmons, who understood that you don't need to be on a smartphone throughout the day to cultivate a readership.

Turning off your smartphone is possible.

It can be comforting to know that there are others who feel the same as you. That there are people who aren't just saying that their phones are negatively impacting their lives but are doing something about it.

When you are watching your kid's soccer game and see other parents on the sidelines looking down at their screens, that doesn't have to be you. When you go to a concert and see the rest of the audience holding their phones in the air to record, you can remind yourself that you have the ability to be present. You have the power to do it—and the first step is to turn off your phone.

This book is your manifesto. It is time to take action.

It's your turn.

Write to Me!

Thank you for reading! I would love to hear about your journey and the strategies you have implemented from the book.

You can email me at author@richard-simon.com. I will read all messages sent to this address, but due to time constraints, I can't promise that I will respond to every message. Good luck!

Acknowledgments

First and foremost, I'm immensely grateful to my wife, Lauren. She was the first person I pitched the idea for my smartphone detox, and she was with me every step of the way on this journey. No one took on more during this five-year stretch than her. I'm grateful for her love and endless support.

My parents and in-laws played a big part in ensuring the success of the book, especially during the writing and editing phases when we needed help with the kids. I'm grateful for their encouragement and love.

When I delivered the manuscript to my editor, the most overwhelming feeling I had was gratitude. From 2021 to 2024, I conducted dozens of interviews with people who were generous enough to share their story with me and allow me to tell it. I am deeply appreciative to each person I interviewed, some of whom didn't end up in the book. Thank you for your time and for sharing your story. I learned a lot from each of you, and I trust that others will too.

The first person I shared my book idea with outside of my immediate family was my former colleague, Anne Cassidy. In the early stages, she provided me with the encouragement I needed to move forward.

Herta Feely helped tremendously as I shaped my book proposal, and this paid off in another way, as it led me to my literary agent, Emily Williamson. Emily was relentless in finding the right home for this book. I'm thankful for all that she has done to make it a success.

The book that you hold today would look very different if it weren't for my editor, John Meils. John's passion for this topic was clear on our first call together, and the overall narrative and words on each page benefited from his guidance. I'm grateful for all his hard work and vision.

I am also grateful to Julia Perry, who helped get this book across the finish line. Her skill as an editor in balancing aggressive deadlines with poise amazed me.

Many thanks to additional members of the Workman team, including Kimberly Ehart and designers Jack Dunnington and Galen Smith. The marketing team was a joy to work with including Moira Kerrigan and Diana Griffin, who passionately promoted the book to a broader audience.

In January 2019, the *Wall Street Journal* profiled Cal Newport in its weekend edition. I remember reading the profile and feeling both comforted and empowered that there was someone else concerned about emerging technology and its impact on our lives. I proceeded to devour Cal's books, and his work continues to inspire me. As I was working on the proposal for this project, Cal and I connected over the phone, and when I told him about my book, he said, "Oh, that will sell." Those words meant a lot to me.

As word got out among friends about what I was writing, I kept hearing the same thing: "I need to read your book" or "My wife/husband needs to read your book." At a certain point, I understood it wasn't just flattery, and that the theme for this book had struck a chord. Many friends offered insights and encouragement along the way, for which I am thankful.

The teachings of Rabbi Daniel Lerner, Rabbi Shmuel Silber, and Rabbi Levi Druk informed my thinking on a number of the ideas in this book. I've grown in my spirituality because of them, and I am grateful for their friendship.

Finally, to Akiva, Hillel, and Miriam. I hope you can pick up this book when you are older and find meaning. Ema and I love you.

Sources

....

Articles

"20 Vital Smartphone Usage Statistics [2022]: Facts + Trends on Mobile Use in the U.S.–Zippia." April 3, 2023. https://www.zippia.com/advice/smartphone-usage-statistics/.

"Charted: There Are More Mobile Phones than People in the World." World Economic Forum, April 11, 2023. https://www.weforum.org/agenda/2023/04/charted-there-are-more-phones-than-people-in-the-world/.

"Chess.com Reaches 100 Million Members." Chess.com, December 16, 2022. https://www.chess.com/article/view/chesscom-reaches-100-million-members.

Dekker, Cynthia A, and Susanne E. Baumgartner. "Is Life Brighter When Your Phone Is Not? The Efficacy of a Grayscale Smartphone Intervention Addressing Digital Well-Being." *Mobile Media & Communication*. 2023. https://doi.org/10.1177/20501579231212062.

"Distracted Driving | Cellphone Use." National Conference of State Legislatures, last updated July 24, 2024. https://www.ncsl.org/transportation/distracted-driving-cellphone-use#:~:text=Nearly%20303%20million%20people%20in.

"The Flip Phone Experiment." *Observer*, October 31, 2022. https://www.ndsmcobserver.com/article/2022/10/the-flip-phone-experiment.

"For the Children's Sake, Put Down That Smartphone," NPR. National Public Radio, April 21, 2014. https://www.npr.org/transcripts/304196338.

"Gen Zers Are Snapping up Flip Phones. They Might Be onto Something." *Wall Street Journal*, May 2, 2023. https://www.wsj.com/articles/gen-z-flip-phones-might-be-onto-something-c4744796.

"Jack White on Immigration, Hating Mobile Phones and His Musical Influences." Channel 4 News, June 19, 2019. https://www.youtube.com/watch?v=LKXQwrjdxOU.

"Patterns of Mobile Device Use by Caregivers and Children during Meals in Fast Food Restaurants." *Pediatrics* 133 (4): e843–49. https://doi.org/10.1542/peds.2013-3703.

Pew Research Center. "Americans and Their Cell Phones." April 3, 2006. https://www.pewresearch.org/internet/2006/04/03/americans-and-their-cell-phones-2/.

Pew Research Center. "Internet and Cell Phone Facts." July 26, 2005. https://www.pewresearch.org/internet/2005/07/26/internet-and-cell-phone-facts/.

Pew Research Center. "Mobile Fact Sheet." January 31, 2024. https://www.pewresearch.org/internet/fact-sheet/mobile/.

Pew Research Center. "Smartphone Adoption and Usage." July 11, 2011. https://www.pewresearch.org/internet/2011/07/11/smartphone-adoption-and-usage/.

"The Phone in the Room." *The New York Times*, February 27, 2023. https://www.nytimes.com/2023/02/27/briefing/phones-mental-health.html.

"A Piece of Advice I Wish I'd Included in My Book." Cal Newport's Study Hacks Blog, October 21, 2019. https://calnewport.com/a-piece-of-advice-i-wish-id-included-in-my-book/.

"Reflections on the Disconnected Life." Cal Newport's Study Hacks Blog, November 24, 2019. https://calnewport.com/reflections-on-the-disconnected-life/

"Smartphones Have Turbocharged the Danger of Porn." *Wall Street Journal*, October 13, 2023. https://www.wsj.com/tech/smartphones-have-turbocharged-the-danger-of-porn-a701eeaf.

"Topic: Smartphone Industry Analysis." Statista, 2018. https://www.statista.com/topics/840/smartphones/.

"Top 10 Smartphone Uses: New Consumer Report Reveals Why We're at the Point of No Return [EmpowerQ]." April 7, 2023. https://www.qualcomm.com/news/onq/2023/04/top-10-smartphone-uses-new-consumer-report-reveals-why-were-at-the-point-of-no-return.

"What the Beep? Die-Hards Refuse to Let Go of Their Pagers." *Wall Street Journal*. May 19, 2023. https://www.wsj.com/articles/still-use-pagers-to-avoid-technology-burnout-1296d6e0.

"Yuck: 88% Use Smartphones on the Toilet, and 44% Put Those Phones in Their Mouths." TechRepublic. https://www.techrepublic.com/article/yuck-88-use-smartphones-on-the-toilet-and-44-put-those-phones-in-their-mouths/.

Books

Alter, Adam L. 2017. *Irresistible: The Rise of Addictive Technology and the Business of Keeping Us Hooked*. Penguin Books.

Bruce, Robert V. 1990. *Bell: Alexander Graham Bell and the Conquest of Solitude*. Ithaca: Cornell University Press.

Goggin, Gerard. 2006. *Cell Phone Culture: Mobile Technology in Everyday Life*. Routledge.

Hassan, Robert. 2019. *Uncontained: Digital Disconnection and the Experience of Time*. Grattan Street Press.

Kagge, Erling. 2019. *Walking: One Step at a Time*. Vintage.

Lembke, Anna, MD. 2023. *Dopamine Nation*. Penguin Random House.

Merchant, Brian. 2017. The One Device: *The Secret History of the iPhone*. Little, Brown and Company.

Newport, Cal. 2018. Deep Work: *Rules for Focused Success in a Distracted World*. Grand Central Publishing.

O'Mara, S. M. 2021. *In Praise of Walking: A New Scientific Exploration*. W. W. Norton & Company.

Southern Telephone News. United States: Southern Bell Telephone and Telegraph Company, Cumberland Telephone and Telegraph Company, Incorporated, 1921.

Turkle, Sherry. 2015. *Reclaiming Conversation: The Power of Talk in a Digital Age*. Penguin Books.